Get Ahead!
Basic Sciences
100 EMQs

Anna Kowalewski
Foundation Doctor, London

Priya Jeevananthan
Obstetric and Gynaecology Registrar
Queen Charlotte's and Chelsea Hospital, London

Series Editor
Saran Shantikumar
Academic Clinical Fellow in Public Health
University of Warwick
Coventry, UK

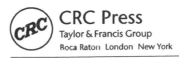

CRC Press
Taylor & Francis Group
Boca Raton London New York

CRC Press is an imprint of the
Taylor & Francis Group, an **informa** business

CRC Press
Taylor & Francis Group
6000 Broken Sound Parkway NW, Suite 300
Boca Raton, FL 33487-2742

© 2017 by Taylor & Francis Group, LLC
CRC Press is an imprint of Taylor & Francis Group, an Informa business

No claim to original U.S. Government works

Printed on acid-free paper
Version Date: 20161017

International Standard Book Number-13: 978-1-4987-5103-2 (Paperback)

Visit the Taylor & Francis Web site at
http://www.taylorandfrancis.com

and the CRC Press Web site at
http://www.crcpress.com

Contents

Preface

Welcome to *Get Ahead! Basic Sciences: 100 EMQs*.

Here is a collection of EMQs to get you started on your road to medical school success! With any exam the key is practice, practice, practice. We cannot emphasise enough how important it is to answer as many questions as you can before your exams. This book, along with its companion volume *Get Ahead! Basic Sciences: 500 SBAs*, is a great way to test your knowledge, whether you are at the start, middle or scarily close to your exams.

The knowledge required to pass your exams is seemingly infinite. As soon as you learn one aspect, a thousand more immediately seem more important. To be a good doctor you have to be a lifelong learner. However, just knowing 'stuff' is not enough. You need to know how to play the game. One way to get yourself ahead is to read as many questions as possible. The more you read, the more you realise the same questions are being asked again and again albeit in slightly different ways. Undergraduate exams are not here to catch you out.

To help your studying, the questions have been organised in two ways. The first three papers have certain topics grouped together to focus your attention on a specific area, for example, the cell or cardiology. In contrast, the last two papers are in an exam style, perfect for using as practice closer to exam time. We would suggest setting a time limit of 40 minutes for each paper, leaving you 2 minutes for each question.

In summary, practice, practice, and practice some more. Good luck.

Anna Kowalewski
Priya Jeevananthan

Contributors

WRITTEN AND EDITED BY
Anna Kowalewski
Priya Jeevananthan

ADDITIONAL CONTRIBUTORS
Neel Sharma
Avishek Das
Pavithra Logitharajah
Chinedu Maduakor
Vikram Malhotra
Ian Mann
John Nehme
Naomi Periselmeris
Donna Pilkington
James Richardson
Ravnita Sharma
Naren Srinivasan
Stephanie Stone
Helen Butler

SERIES EDITOR
Saran Shantikumar

EMQs Paper 1

1. CARDIOLOGY

A. Aortic regurgitation
B. Aortic stenosis
C. Mitral regurgitation
D. Mitral stenosis
E. Pulmonary regurgitation
F. Pulmonary stenosis
G. Tricuspid regurgitation
H. Tricuspid stenosis

For each of the following scenarios, select the most appropriate condition. Each option may be used once, more than once or not at all.

1. A 58-year-old male patient presents with a history of exertional chest pain and dizziness. He notices he becomes short of breath on climbing stairs.
2. A 70-year-old female patient has a 'bobbing uvula' and an early diastolic murmur best heard at the left sternal edge, 4th intercostal space on examination.
3. A 44-year-old female patient presents to her GP with palpitations and is found to be in atrial fibrillation. Further questioning reveals a history of 'a jerking movement disorder' as a child. She is found to have a murmur and facial flushing on examination.
4. A 76-year-old male patient has a loud pansystolic murmur and lateral displacement of his apex beat. The murmur is heard best with the breath held in full expiration.
5. A 24-year-old male patient of no fixed abode presents to accident and emergency with a high temperature and looks unwell. He has a pansystolic murmur heard best on inspiration. Multiple scars are observed over his arms, and it is especially difficult to find a vein to cannulate.

2. PHARMACOLOGY

A. Angiotensin-converting enzyme inhibitors
B. Beta-blockers
C. Calcium channel blockers
D. Loop diuretics
E. Methyldopa
F. Minoxidil

G. Potassium sparing diuretics

H. Thiazide diuretics

For each of the following scenarios, select the most appropriate medication. Each option may be used once, more than once or not at all.

1. A male patient has started on a drug by his GP and now reports problems sustaining erections.
2. A female patient has developed a swollen, tender first metatarsophalangeal joint in her left foot since starting this new medication.
3. A male patient has started on a new medication as an inpatient for severe hypertension by a specialist. He notices that his male-pattern balding seems to be improving with the growth of new hair.
4. A female patient has developed a dry irritating cough after starting a new medication.
5. A male patient has developed constipation and ankle swelling after starting this drug.

3. CARDIOLOGY

A. Collapsing pulse

B. Electrical alternans

C. Jerky pulse

D. Pulsus alternans

E. Pulsus bisferiens

F. Pulsus paradoxus

G. Radial femoral delay

H. Slow rising pulse

For each of the following scenarios, select the most appropriate examination finding. Each option may be used once, more than once or not at all.

1. A 66-year-old female patient reveals a wide pulse pressure and an early diastolic murmur.
2. An 82-year-old male patient is found to have a loud ejection systolic murmur radiating to the carotids. What else would you expect to find?
3. A 24-year-old male student with a family history of sudden unexplained death at a young age presents with dizzy spells and occasional palpitations. Examination reveals a double apical impulse. What else might be found on examination?
4. A 21-year-old female patient has a wide carrying angle and an abnormal chest X-ray. The X-ray shows a normal heart size but some rib notching. Which sign may you expect to find on examination?
5. A 76-year-old male patient is known to have severe left ventricular failure. On palpation of the carotid pulse you notice the volume does not feel the same each time.

4. CARDIOLOGY

A. Atrial flutter with 2:1 block
B. Atrial flutter with 3:1 block
C. Bifascicular block
D. Complete heart block
E. First-degree heart block
F. Mobitz type I heart block
G. Mobitz type II heart block
H. Trifascicular block

For each of the following descriptions, select the most appropriate ECG pattern. Each option may be used once, more than once or not at all.

1. A ventricular rate of 100 beats per minute with a saw-tooth appearance between the R–R intervals.
2. Sinus rhythm with normal axis, a QRS duration of 96 ms and a PR interval of 238 ms.
3. Sinus rhythm, left axis deviation, a QRS duration of 110 ms with a right bundle branch block pattern and a PR interval of 230 ms.
4. Ventricular rate of 40 beats per minute, and P-waves at a rate of 90 beats per minute which seem to 'march through' the trace.
5. A prolonged PR interval followed by a 'dropped beat'. The PR then resets and the cycle repeats.

5. CARDIOLOGY

A. Aorta
B. Circumflex artery
C. Diagonal artery
D. Left anterior descending artery
E. Left main stem
F. Obtuse marginal artery
G. Posterior descending artery
H. Right coronary artery

For each of the following descriptions, select the most appropriate artery. Each option may be used once, more than once or not at all.

1. This runs in the anterior interventricular groove.
2. This supplies the sinoatrial node (SAN) in 60% of individuals.
3. Inferior ischaemic changes on the ECG in the context of aortic dissection are likely to involve this coronary artery.
4. This runs in the posterior interventricular sulcus.
5. This is a branch of the circumflex artery and travels towards the apex of the heart.

6. RESPIRATORY

A. Aortic arch
B. Bulbopontine controller
C. Carotid body
D. Golgi tendon organs
E. Irritant receptors
F. J receptors
G. Medulla chemoreceptor
H. Suprapontine controller
I. None of the above

For each of the following descriptions, select the most appropriate part of the respiratory tract. Each option may be used once, more than once or not at all.

1. This is responsible for automatic respiratory drive.
2. These lie between airway epithelial cells and are stimulated by mechanical stimuli.
3. This is responsible for wilful control of respiratory drive.
4. A chemoreceptor that is able to detect pH.
5. A chemoreceptor that is able to detect $PaCO_2$ but not arterial pH or hypoxia.

7. RESPIRATORY SYSTEM (LOWER): ANATOMY AND PHYSIOLOGY

A. Expiratory capacity
B. Expiratory reserve volume
C. Functional residual capacity
D. Inspiratory capacity
E. Inspiratory reserve volume
F. Residual volume
G. Tidal volume
H. Total lung capacity
I. Vital capacity

For each of the following descriptions, select the most appropriate lung volume or capacity. Each option may be used once, more than once or not at all.

1. This volume is approximately 500 mL in an average healthy adult.
2. The volume of air that can be breathed in on maximal inspiration, at the end of normal inspiration.
3. The volume of air that can be breathed in on maximal inspiration from a baseline of maximal expiration.
4. This volume is approximately 3800 mL in an average healthy adult.
5. The volume of air that remains in the lungs after quiet expiration.

8. RESPIRATORY SYSTEM (LOWER): ANATOMY AND PHYSIOLOGY

A. Chief cells
B. Clara cells
C. Fibrous cartilage
D. Goblet cells
E. Hyaline cartilage
F. Parietal cells
G. Smooth muscle cells
H. Type II pneumocytes

For each of the following descriptions, select the most appropriate type of cell or cartilage. Each option may be used once, more than once or not at all.

1. Allow the physiological response of airways to hypoxia.
2. Provide structural integrity to the airways.
3. Secrete mucus.
4. Secrete protein-rich fluid.
5. Produce surfactant.

9. RESPIRATORY

A. Choanal atresia
B. Cystic fibrosis
C. Kartagener syndrome
D. Laryngocoele
E. Laryngomalacia
F. Mounier–Kuhn syndrome
G. Tracheomalacia
H. Tracheostenosis
I. None of the above

For each of the following descriptions, select the most appropriate diagnosis. Each option may be used once, more than once or not at all.

1. A disorder of the cilia lining the respiratory tract.
2. The result of immature cartilage leading to the collapse of the upper larynx during inhalation.
3. A congenital anomalous air sac which communicates with the cavity of the larynx.
4. A complication of Wegener's granulomatosis.
5. The congenital disorder in which one or both of the nasal passages are blocked by soft or bony tissue.

10. RESPIRATORY

A. Air
B. Bilevel positive airway pressure (BiPAP)

C. Continuous positive airway pressure (CPAP)
D. Nasal cannulae
E. Reservoir bag mask
F. Simple face mask
G. Venturi mask
H. None of the above

For each of the following descriptions, select the most appropriate delivery system or treatment. Each option may be used once, more than once or not at all.

1. This can accurately deliver 24% oxygen to a patient.
2. This consistently provides 20% oxygen to a patient.
3. This contains a simple one-way valve.
4. This can only comfortably provide oxygen at low flow rates.
5. This can be used in severe obstructive sleep apnoea.

11. THE CELL

A. Apoptosis
B. Clonal expansion
C. Hyperplasia
D. Hypertrophy
E. Meiosis
F. Mitosis
G. Necrosis
H. Neoplasia

For each of the following, select the most appropriate cellular process. Each option may be used once, more than once or not at all.

1. The process in which membrane blebbing occurs.
2. The process in which there is disruption of organelles.
3. The process in which there is lysosomal spillage.
4. The process in which tissue transglutaminase plays a role.
5. The process in which a tissue increases in size as the number of cells increases.

12. THE CELL

A. G0
B. G1
C. G2
D. G3
E. G4
F. M phase
G. *RB* checkpoint
H. S phase

For each of the following, select the most appropriate cellular process. Each option may be used once, more than once or not at all.

1. Name the stage of the cell cycle in which mitosis occurs.
2. Name the stage of the cell cycle where the two daughter cells are formed.
3. Name the stage where cell replication does *not* occur.
4. Name the stage at which genome replication and DNA synthesis occur.
5. Name the stage at which the chromosomes are prepared for replication.

13. THE CELL

A. Golgi apparatus
B. Mitochondria
C. Nuclear envelope
D. Nuclear pore
E. Nucleolus
F. Rough endoplasmic reticulum
G. Smooth endoplasmic reticulum
H. None of the above

For each of the following descriptions, select the most appropriate part of the nucleus or cell. Each option may be used once, more than once or not at all.

1. This is studded with ribosomes which are used for protein synthesis.
2. This has a major function in lipid metabolism.
3. This is involved in the modification of macromolecules before secretion.
4. This provides support to the nucleus.
5. This assembles ribosomes.

14. ACID–BASE BALANCE

A. Metabolic acidosis
B. Metabolic acidosis with compensation
C. Metabolic alkalosis
D. No effect
E. Respiratory acidosis
F. Respiratory acidosis with compensation
G. Respiratory alkalosis
H. None of the above

For each of the following descriptions, select the most commonly associated acid–base imbalance. Each option may be used once, more than once or not at all.

1. Insufflation during laparoscopy
2. Anxiety attack
3. Malignant hyperthermia
4. Opiate overdose
5. Cardiac arrest

15. ACID–BASE BALANCE

A. pH 6.9 and PCO_2 8.4 kPa
B. pH 7.17 and PCO_2 3.1 kPa
C. pH 7.22 and PCO_2 3.9 kPa
D. pH 7.30 and PCO_2 7.3 kPa
E. pH 7.49 and PCO_2 5.4 kPa
F. pH 7.54 and PCO_2 3.7 kPa
G. pH 7.66 and PCO_2 7.4 kPa
H. None of the above

For each of the following scenarios, select the most appropriate arterial blood gas values. Each option may be used once, more than once or not at all.

1. A 13-year-old boy with cystic fibrosis has a new cough productive of green sputum, which has developed over the past few days. He is now complaining of shortness of breath.
2. A 67-year-old man presents after complaining of left-sided chest pain to his wife only 1 hour earlier. He requires resuscitation. He is now on oxygen.
3. A 78-year-old woman suffered a severe stroke and was intubated. She is now in the intensive care unit. It was noted that she had been hyperventilating.
4. A 20-year-old medical student ate a rather dubious kebab and has vomited up to 20 times over the past few days and has been not been able to eat. His friend took an arterial blood gas for practice.
5. A 19-year-old non-compliant insulin-dependent diabetic man was admitted after feeling his breathing was becoming abnormal.

16. HAEMATOLOGY

A. B lymphocytes
B. Basophils
C. Eosinophils
D. Monocytes
E. Natural killer cells
F. Neutrophils
G. Plasma cells
H. T lymphocytes

For each of the following descriptions, select the most appropriate cell type. Each option may be used once, more than once or not at all.

1. These are responsible for cell-mediated immunity.
2. These are otherwise known as acidophils.
3. These migrate to sites of injury and discharge their histamine-containing granules.
4. These are important in preventing cancer.
5. These are specialized to synthesize and secrete antibodies.

17. HAEMATOLOGY

A. Aplastic anaemia
B. β-Thalassaemia
C. Blood loss anaemia
D. Haemolytic anaemia
E. Megaloblastic anaemia
F. Polycythaemia vera
G. Secondary polycythaemia
H. Sickle cell anaemia

For each of the following descriptions, select the most appropriate condition. Each option may be used once, more than once or not at all.

1. This is caused by dietary folate deficiency.
2. This is caused by abnormal beta-chains of the haemoglobin molecule.
3. This can result from exposure to gamma ray radiation from a nuclear bomb.
4. This is caused by hereditary spherocytosis.
5. This can occur after rapid haemorrhage secondary to trauma.

18. HAEMATOLOGY

A. B-cells
B. Basophils
C. Megaloblastic cells
D. Normal red cells
E. Platelets
F. Plasma cells
G. T-cells
H. Target cells

For each of the following descriptions, select the most appropriate cell type. Each option may be used once, more than once or not at all.

1. These cells are produced in the bone marrow from megakaryocytes.
2. These cells do not have a nucleus.
3. These cells are released into the circulation as immature cells called reticulocytes.
4. These cells may be seen in folate deficiency.
5. These cells produce antibodies.

19. HAEMATOLOGY

A. Calcium
B. Factor V
C. Factor X
D. Factor Xa
E. Factor XIIa

F. Factor XIIIa
G. Fibrinogen
H. Platelet phospholipid
I. Stable fibrin
J. Thrombin
K. Tissue thromboplastin

For each of the following descriptions, select the most appropriate term. Each option may be used once, more than once or not at all.

1. This is part of the intrinsic pathway.
2. This is part of the extrinsic pathway.
3. This is activated by both the intrinsic and extrinsic pathways.
4. This converts fibrin into a stable fibrin clot.
5. This activates factor XIII.

20. HAEMATOLOGY

A. PT: ↑   APTT: ↑   TT: ↔/↑   Platelets: ↓
B. PT: ↑   APTT: ↑   TT: ↑   Platelets: ↓
C. PT: ↓   APTT: ↑   TT: ↔/↑   Platelets: ↓
D. PT: ↑   APTT: ↑   TT: ↔   Platelets: ↔
E. PT: ↑   APTT: ↑   TT: ↑   Platelets: ↔
F. PT: ↓   APTT: ↑   TT: ↑   Platelets: ↔

For each of the following disorders, select the most appropriate coagulation changes that would occur. Each option may be used once, more than once or not at all. Abbreviations are as follows: PT (prothrombin time); APTT (activated partial thrombin time); TT (thrombin time); ↔ (normal); ↑ (increased); ↓ (decreased).

1. Liver disease
2. Heparin
3. Massive transfusion
4. Vitamin K deficiency
5. Disseminated intravascular coagulation (DIC)

Answers Paper 1

ANSWER QUESTION 1

1. B – Aortic stenosis

This is a typical presentation of what is likely to be critical aortic stenosis. Due to this patient's age, the most likely cause of his aortic stenosis is going to be a congenital bicuspid aortic valve. The normal aortic valve should comprise three cusps. Up to 2% of the population are born with a bicuspid aortic valve, and they are prone to premature calcification and subsequent stenosis. Patients with aortic stenosis typically become symptomatic on exertion as the myocardial oxygen requirements increase; however, the stenotic aortic valve prevents adequate perfusion of the coronary arteries.

2. A – Aortic regurgitation

Aortic regurgitation is heard as an early diastolic murmur, best auscultated by leaning the patient forward with the breath held in expiration. Place the diaphragm of the stethoscope on the left sternal edge, 4th intercostal space. There are many eponymous signs associated with aortic regurgitation. The 'bobbing uvula' in this case is called Müller's sign. It occurs during systole secondary to an increased stroke volume.

3. D – Mitral stenosis

This patient has mitral stenosis, which is almost always associated with a history of rheumatic fever. It is the mitral valve that is affected in more than 90% of cases of rheumatic fever, and mitral stenosis is more prevalent in women. A low-pitched rumbling mid-diastolic murmur is characteristic. Patients with mitral stenosis are commonly in atrial fibrillation as they have a dilated left atrium. The childhood movement disorder that is described in the scenario is the clue to a history of rheumatic fever. This is known as Sydenham's chorea (a.k.a. Saint Vitus Dance) and occurs in approximately 10% of patients who suffer with rheumatic fever.

4. C – Mitral regurgitation

This is a classic description of mitral regurgitation, which is commonly found in clinical practice. The pansystolic murmur can be differentiated from the pansystolic murmur of tricuspid regurgitation by holding the breath in different phases of the respiratory cycle. Murmurs of the right heart will be accentuated by held inspiration (increased venous return), and murmurs of the left heart by held expiration (increases flow to the left side of the heart).

5. G – Tricuspid regurgitation

There are several clues as to the underlying pathology in this patient. He is an intravenous drug user (IVDU). The clues to this are the scars on his arms and the difficulty in finding a vein for cannulation. His temperature, combined with a cardiac murmur, arouses suspicion of endocarditis. He has a pansystolic murmur which is right-sided, as it is accentuated on inspiration. IVDU patients are at increased risk of right heart endocarditis and it is commonly the tricuspid valve that is affected.

ANSWER QUESTION 2

1. B – Beta-blockers

Beta-blockers quite commonly result in difficulty sustaining erections. Other common side-effects are hallucinations, nightmares and vivid dreams. They are also associated with depressed mood, hypotension and poor exercise effort. All side-effects are reversed on withdrawal of the medication.

2. H – Thiazide diuretics

Thiazide diuretics can precipitate acute gout, with the first metatarsophalangeal joint being the most commonly affected. Thiazide diuretics work by the inhibition of sodium absorption at the beginning of the distal convoluted tubule. Other common adverse effects include dehydration, hyponatraemia, hypokalaemia, hypercalcaemia and occasionally impotence.

3. F – Minoxidil

Minoxidil is not commonly used for hypertension; however, it is extremely useful for patients with severe hypertension requiring inpatient control. This drug is a potent antihypertensive which exerts its effects through vasodilation. Minoxidil is given as a continuous intravenous infusion and patients should be weaned off slowly. Abruptly stopping minoxidil can result in rebound hypertension.

4. A – Angiotensin-converting enzyme inhibitors

ACE inhibitors can cause a dry cough in around 20% of patients. The mechanism, although not fully understood, is thought to be due to increased alveolar and bronchiolar concentrations of bradykinin, which stimulates cough receptors.

5. C – Calcium channel blockers

Calcium channel blockers can commonly result in ankle swelling, headaches and constipation. Ankle swelling is particularly common with the dihydropyridine calcium channel blockers such as amlodipine and nifedipine.

ANSWER QUESTION 3

1. A – Collapsing pulse
The murmur described is that of aortic regurgitation. An associated finding is a wide pulse pressure. This is due to the regurgitant flow lowering the aortic diastolic pressure. A collapsing pulse, in either a carotid artery or a peripheral limb artery, is an associated examination finding that may also be present with arteriovenous fistulae, patent ductus arteriosus or other large extracardiac shunts. On occasion, an Austin Flint murmur may also be heard in conjunction with aortic regurgitation. This is a mid-diastolic murmur of the mitral valve caused by the regurgitant jet of blood from the aortic valve striking the anterior mitral valve leaflet.

2. H – Slow rising pulse
A slow rising pulse is associated with aortic stenosis. Other features of aortic stenosis are a narrow pulse pressure, a double apical impulse and a systolic thrill over the aortic valve area. The age of a patient may give you clues as to the cause of the aortic stenosis.

3. C – Jerky pulse
The description is of a family history of sudden cardiac death in a patient with presyncopal symptoms and palpitations. This is likely to be hypertrophic obstructive cardiomyopathy (HOCM). The characteristic pulse is said to be of a 'jerky' nature. Other clinical findings are a large *a* wave in the jugular venous pressure, a double apical impulse, an ejection systolic murmur and often paradoxical splitting of the second heart sound.

4. G – Radial femoral delay
The history is of a patient with Turner syndrome. Affected patients have a wide carrying angle, widely spaced nipples and a webbed neck. Turner syndrome is associated with aortic coarctation. A chest X-ray may show a normal heart size and rib notching (caused by the pulsation of dilated intercostal arteries). Aortic coarctation is associated with the clinical finding of radial–femoral delay.

5. D – Pulsus alternans
Pulsus alternans is a sign of severe left ventricular failure. Palpation of the pulse will reveal alternating strong and weak beats. It is associated with a poor prognosis. Electrical alternans is completely different. This is where the electrical axis or QRS amplitude alternates between beats on the ECG and is found in cardiac tamponade.

ANSWER QUESTION 4

1. B – Atrial flutter with 3:1 block
Atrial flutter is commonly referred to as having a 'saw-tooth' appearance on an ECG. This is a macro re-entry circuit, which can be easily DC (direct current) cardioverted. The ventricular rate is important in determining

the level of the block, and flutter is characterised by an atrial contraction rate of 300 per minute. A ventricular rate of 100 beats per minute signifies a 3:1 block (i.e. every third atrial beat is conducted to the ventricles), and a ventricular rate of 150 beats per minute signifies a 2:1 block.

2. E – First-degree heart block

The normal PR interval should be less than 210 ms, and in this case it is prolonged at 238 ms. In itself this is perfectly benign and is extremely common, particularly in the ageing population. Occasionally patients with a first-degree heart block may become symptomatic; however, this is not especially common.

3. H – Trifascicular block

Trifascicular block is characterised by a prolonged PR interval (first-degree heart block), right bundle branch block and either a left posterior or left anterior fascicular block (with left axis deviation). After the bundle of His, the fibres divide into the left and right bundles. The left bundle further divides into the anterior and posterior fascicles. The combination of a prolonged PR interval (first-degree heart block) with left axis deviation and right bundle branch is said to be a 'trifascicular block'. Patients may require pacing.

4. D – Complete heart block

It is important to know about intrinsic nodal rates to understand the physiology behind this. The SAN has an intrinsic pacemaker rate of between 60 and 100 per minute. The atrioventricular node (AVN) controls the rate at which ventricular contraction occurs and has an intrinsic firing rate of 40–60 per minute. In complete heart block there is complete atrioventricular dissociation, which results in both the ventricles and atria pacing at their own intrinsic rates.

5. F – Mobitz type I heart block

Mobitz type I (also known as Wenckebach) heart block is characterized by progressive prolonging of the PR interval until there is a P-wave with no conducted ventricular (QRS) complex. The cycle resets. This does not usually require a pacemaker. Mobitz type II heart blocks have a risk of developing into a complete heart block and is an indication for a pacemaker.

ANSWER QUESTION 5

1. D – Left anterior descending artery
Occlusions of the left anterior descending artery result in anterior ST changes.

2. H – Right coronary artery
The right coronary artery supplies the SAN in 60% of people. The other 40% derive the blood supply to the SAN from the left circumflex artery.

3. H – Right coronary artery
The right coronary artery can be involved in aortic dissection. This will result in inferior ECG changes. The left main stem may also be affected; however, this would produce anterior changes on the ECG.

4. G – Posterior descending artery
The posterior descending artery runs in the posterior interventricular sulcus. Occlusions will result in posterior infarcts.

5. F – Obtuse marginal artery
The obtuse marginal artery is a branch of the circumflex which runs towards the apex.

ANSWER QUESTION 6

1. B – Bulbopontine controller
2. E – Irritant receptors
3. H – Suprapontine controller
4. C – Carotid body
5. G – Medulla chemoreceptor

Automatic respiratory drive is provided by the bulbopontine area, whereas wilful drive is by the suprapontine area. Suprapontine control can be learned, for example in speaking or playing an instrument, and because it is learned it competes for the control of the respiratory muscles. Irritant receptors lie between the epithelial cells to detect mechanical stimuli such as smoke. They are more sensitive to mechanical irritants and are less sensitive to chemical irritants in the central airways, and vice versa for the more peripheral airways. Note that they are also sensitive to histamine and can compound bronchoconstriction. Juxtacapillary (J) receptors are present within the alveolar walls and are consequently in close contact with the capillaries. They respond to an increase in fluid within the lung parenchyma. Carotid and aortic bodies make up the peripheral chemoreceptors. pH is detected only by carotid bodies, whereas both the carotid and aortic bodies detect changes in blood oxygen and carbon dioxide. Central chemoreceptors are located on the surface of the medulla and respond only to changes in $PaCO_2$.

ANSWER QUESTION 7

1. G – Tidal volume
Tidal volume – the volume of air inhaled or exhaled in a single normal breath – is about 500 mL in an average healthy adult.

2. E – Inspiratory reserve volume
The inspiratory reserve volume is about 3300 mL. The inspiratory reserve volume together with the normal inspiratory volume is called the inspiratory capacity.

3. I – Vital capacity

Vital capacity is the volume of air that can be breathed in on maximal inspiration from a baseline of maximal expiration. This is about 4800 mL in the average non-diseased adult lung. It is the sum of tidal volume and both inspiratory and expiratory reserve capacities.

4. D – Inspiratory capacity

The inspiratory capacity is the sum of tidal volume and inspiratory reserve volume, and signifies the total volume of air that can be breathed in at the end of normal expiration.

5. C – Functional residual capacity

The functional residual capacity (FRC) is about 2200 mL in an average healthy adult. It differs from the residual volume in that residual volume is the amount of air left in the lungs after maximal expiration. FRC is thus the sum of residual volume and expiratory reserve volume.

ANSWER QUESTION 8

1. G – Smooth muscle cells

The physiological response of the airways to hypoxia is bronchoconstriction. This diverts ventilation to areas of the lung that have a better blood supply, thus maintaining a good V/Q (ventilation:perfusion) ratio. This bronchoconstriction is mediated by smooth muscle cells in the airways.

2. E – Hyaline cartilage

Hyaline cartilage lines the trachea as discontinuous rings and also provides structural integrity to the bronchi in the form of flat plates of cartilage. The cartilaginous support ensures that the airways do not collapse after expiration.

3. D – Goblet cells

Goblet cells secrete mucus. Mucus production is an integral part of the mucociliary clearance defence mechanism of the airways.

4. B – Clara cells

Clara cells are non-ciliated cells that secrete protein-rich fluid which are an important part of the lung's defence mechanism.

5. H – Type II pneumocytes

Type II pneumocytes produce surfactant. Surfactant is a lipoprotein lining the alveoli and acts to reduce surface tension.

ANSWER QUESTION 9

1. C – Kartagener syndrome
2. E – Laryngomalacia
3. D – Laryngocoele
4. H – Tracheostenosis
5. A – Choanal atresia

Primary ciliary dyskinesia (PCD, also known as Kartagener syndrome) is a rare autosomal recessive disease in which the respiratory and fallopian cilia are defective. Normally cilia will beat up to 22 times a second but this is significantly decreased in PCD, which leads to poor mucociliary clearance and subsequent respiratory infections. Laryngomalacia is a common condition of infancy where the cartilage is immature and therefore soft. This means that the pressure caused by inspiration will cause the larynx to collapse, leading to airway obstruction. With time, the cartilage will harden and the disorder will disappear. It can also occur in patients with neuromuscular conditions. A laryngocoele is usually a congenital anomalous air sac which communicates with the cavity of the larynx. It can also be seen in patients with chronic obstructive pulmonary disease. Wegener granulomatosis may cause tracheostenosis (tracheal narrowing). Choanal atresia is a congenital condition in which the choanae (the openings at the back of the nasal passages) are blocked by abnormal bony or soft tissue growths during foetal development.

ANSWER QUESTION 10

1. G – Venturi mask
2. A – Air
3. E – Reservoir bag mask
4. D – Nasal cannulae
5. C – Continuous positive airway pressure (CPAP)

The concentration of oxygen at sea level is 21%. A Venturi mask is able to increase the accuracy of oxygen therapy between 24 and 40%, which is useful in chronic obstructive pulmonary disease (COPD) patients with a hypercapnoeic respiratory drive. Nasal cannulae are only comfortable at low flow rates and consequently can only deliver up to 50% oxygen. A non-rebreather or reservoir mask allows the exhaled gas to pass out of the mask but lets the reservoir stay full of oxygen, allowing delivery of almost 80% oxygen. CPAP is used in obstructive sleep apnoeic patients as it keeps the airways patent.

ANSWER QUESTION 11

1. A – Apoptosis
Apoptosis is the process of programmed cell death and is a normal part of growth and development. The process of apoptosis occurs in the following stages:

- Initiation (e.g. deprivation of survival factors, anticancer drugs, irradiation, pro-apoptotic cytokines)
- Membrane blebbing
- Cellular and organelle shrinkage

- DNA condensation and fragmentation
- Phagocytosis of cellular debris

2. G – Necrosis

Necrosis is a pathological process initiated by an external stimulus (e.g. toxins or ischaemia). Unlike apoptosis, it is associated with non-physiological circumstances that disrupt homeostasis. Cellular contents, including degradative enzymes, are spilled out into the tissue and cause necrosis of surrounding cells. It also initiates an inflammatory response which is pathological in itself, causing further tissue damage.

3. G – Necrosis

Necrosis and apoptosis are two forms of cell death. However, there are many differences. Apoptosis is regulated and genetically determined, while necrosis occurs in response to pathological stimuli. Necrosis results in the spillage of internal cellular materials including degradative lysosomes, which damages neighbouring tissue. Types of necrosis include caseous necrosis (central 'cheesy' area, as seen in tuberculosis), liquefaction necrosis (e.g. abscess formation) and coagulation necrosis (e.g. myocardial infarction).

4. A – Apoptosis

Apoptosis can be induced internally, via the mitochondrial pathway, externally, via the death receptor pathway, or via an inducing factor (e.g. chemotherapeutic drugs). It is also known as cell suicide. Advantages over necrosis are the lack of an inflammatory response, there is no spill of cell content and the debris is engulfed by phagocytosis. Apoptosis is a normal part of embryogenesis and growth, and inhibition of apoptotic factors can lead to malignant growth.

5. C – Hyperplasia

Hypertrophy and hyperplasia are often confused. Hypertrophy is an increase in tissue or organ size as a result of an increase in the size of each cell, whereas hyperplasia results in an increased size because of an increased number of constituent cells. Examples of hypertrophy include myocardial hypertrophy. Left ventricular hypertrophy occurs in response to aortic stenosis because of the extra work required to overcome the obstruction. Benign prostatic hyperplasia is an example in which the number of cells increases; it is common in older age probably because of lifelong exposure to testosterone, stimulating cell growth.

ANSWER QUESTION 12

1. F – M phase

Mitosis occurs during the 'M stage' of the cell cycle with the formation of two daughter cells. The new cells can enter into the G0 phase and differentiate into specialized cells, or enter into the cell cycle, which is stimulated by the action of growth factors.

2. F – M phase

The two daughter cells are formed during the 'M stage' when mitosis occurs. Mitosis is the process by which cellular DNA is replicated and separated into two identical nuclei. The two nuclei separate to become part of two identical cells in the process of cytokinesis. Mitosis itself is made up of five stages: interphase, prophase, metaphase, anaphase and telophase.

3. A – G0

G0 is a non-replication phase. A new cell can enter into G0 and undergo differentiation into specialized cells, rather than undergoing replication. Alternatively, it can enter into the cell cycle and replicate further.

4. H – S phase

Genome replication and DNA synthesis occur during the 'S phase'. During this stage, any DNA defects are detected and the cycle is halted via the actions of *TP53*. *TP53* is a protein involved in the control of the cell cycle and apoptosis. Malignancy results from a mutation in *TP53*. For example, colorectal, lung, brain and breast carcinomas have all been associated with mutations in *TP53*. *TP53* halts the cell cycle and induces apoptosis if DNA defects are found.

5. B – G1

G1 is the preparation phase in which proteins that are necessary for protein synthesis are transcribed. After G1, the cell reaches a 'checkpoint' in which the cells with DNA defects undergo apoptosis. Continuation of the cell cycle is inhibited by tumour suppressor genes *RB* and *TP53*, thus mutations of these genes predispose to malignancy.

ANSWER QUESTION 13

1. F – Rough endoplasmic reticulum
2. G – Smooth endoplasmic reticulum
3. A – Golgi apparatus
4. H – None of the above
5. E – Nucleolus

The nucleus is a membrane-enclosed organelle which contains most of a cell's genetic material. The nucleus is enclosed by the nuclear envelope which is a double membrane separating the entire organelle from the rest of the cell. The nuclear lamina is made from two networks of intermediate filaments which provide the nucleus with mechanical support. The inner face is organized, whereas the outer cytosolic face is less organized. Nuclear pores provide the aqueous channels through which molecules of up to 9 nm wide may pass. This size prevents the nuclear material from exiting.

The nucleolus is a discrete densely stained structure which is not surrounded by a separate membrane. It forms around the tandem repeats of rDNA and is able to synthesize rRNA and assemble ribosomes.

In addition to the nucleolus there are other subnuclear bodies including the Cajal bodies, paraspeckles and splicing speckles. The Golgi apparatus processes and packages macromolecules such as proteins for their subsequent secretion or use within the cell. It is composed of membrane bound stacks of cisternae which carry the Golgi enzymes. It has five functional regions: the cis-Golgi network, cis-Golgi, medial-Golgi, trans-Golgi and trans-Golgi network. The vesicles from the endoplasmic reticulum are able to fuse with the cis-Golgi network and progress to the trans-Golgi where they are correctly packaged. This occurs via the vesicular–tubular cluster which mediates the traffic between the endoplasmic reticulum and Golgi. The endoplasmic reticulum is an interconnected network which has several different functions, depending upon the type, but is able (amongst other functions) to provide a place for ribosomes to produce protein.

ANSWER QUESTION 14

1. E – Respiratory acidosis
During laparoscopy the abdomen is insufflated with carbon dioxide. This provides an increased intra-abdominal space in which to work, which helps avoid complications caused by accidental trauma to organs. Abdominal insufflation should only transiently lower the pH.

2. G – Respiratory alkalosis
Overbreathing during an anxiety attack will lead to an excess loss of carbon dioxide. This results in a respiratory alkalosis. In order to compensate, H^+ ions dissociate from circulating albumin, and free Ca^{2+} ions take their place, thus reducing the free calcium concentration. Hence overbreathing can be associated with the symptoms of acute hypocalcaemia, such as peripheral paraesthesia, muscle cramps and tetany.

3. E – Respiratory acidosis
In malignant hyperthermia there is an increase in the production of carbon dioxide from an uncontrolled increase in skeletal muscle metabolism. The acidosis begins as respiratory but will become mixed if not diagnosed quickly.

4. E – Respiratory acidosis
Opiate overdose depresses the respiratory centre and leads to carbon dioxide retention. That is, breathing will slow down and consequently carbon dioxide will stay in the body, leading to a decrease in pH.

5. A – Metabolic acidosis
Cardiac arrest results in impaired tissue perfusion. The subsequent increase in anaerobic respiration and build-up of lactate results in a metabolic acidosis.

ANSWER QUESTION 15

1. D – pH 7.30 and PCO$_2$ 7.3 kPa
This boy has a chest infection, which would cause his breathing and gas exchange to be suboptimal. Consequently, production of carbon dioxide occurs, resulting in a respiratory acidosis.

2. C – pH 7.22 and PCO$_2$ 3.9 kPa
This patient has probably had a myocardial infarction, which will lead to a state of primary metabolic acidosis. Note that this has begun to be compensated for by hyperventilation through cardiopulmonary resuscitation (CPR), hence the low carbon dioxide measurement.

3. F – pH 7.54 and PCO$_2$ 3.7 kPa
This patient is suffering from hyperventilation, causing a decrease in her carbon dioxide levels leading to a respiratory alkalosis.

4. E – pH 7.49 and PCO$_2$ 5.4 kPa
The vomiting will result in the loss of hydrogen ions, thus causing a metabolic alkalosis. Occasionally, some alkaline salts are lost with vomiting, such as bicarbonate, which would result in a mild metabolic acidosis.

5. B – pH 7.17 and PCO$_2$ 3.1 kPa
This patient is suffering from a diabetic ketoacidosis. He has a metabolic acidosis and the body is trying to compensate with Kussmaul (deep and laboured) breathing. This is a medical emergency.

ANSWER QUESTION 16

1. H – T lymphocytes
T lymphocytes are required for cell-mediated immunity, for example involving phagocytosis and cytokine release, while B lymphocytes are required for humoral immunity (e.g. antibody and complement mediated).

2. C – Eosinophils
Eosinophils take up the red dye eosin readily. Eosin is an acidic dye. Acidophil means 'acid loving'.

3. B – Basophils
Basophils contain histamine granules which are released at sites of injury. Histamine causes blood vessel dilation.

4. E – Natural killer cells
Natural killer cells play a role in cancer prevention, having an ability to bind to some tumour and virus-infected cells without prior antigen stimulation. Natural killer cells destroy target cells by first inserting the pore-forming granules (perforin) into the cell membrane, and then releasing granzymes (proteases) which passively diffuse into the target cells and result in apoptosis.

5. A – B lymphocytes

B lymphocytes are white blood cells which secrete antibodies to fight infection.

ANSWER QUESTION 17

1. E – Megaloblastic anaemia

Megaloblasts are very large cells with odd shapes and are found in cases of vitamin B_{12} and folic acid deficiency.

2. H – Sickle cell anaemia

Abnormal haemoglobin S exists in sickle cell anaemia. This is caused by abnormal beta-chains of the haemoglobin molecule.

3. A – Aplastic anaemia

Aplastic anaemia indicates that there is a lack of functioning bone marrow.

4. D – Haemolytic anaemia

Hereditary spherocytosis is an autosomal dominant condition that results in small, spherical erythrocytes. Such red blood cells are extremely fragile and prone to rupture, with an increased rate of degradation in the spleen, resulting in a haemolytic anaemia.

5. C – Blood loss anaemia

Acute blood loss such as that which occurs after major trauma can be rapid, resulting in a severe anaemia requiring blood and blood product transfusion.

ANSWER QUESTION 18

1. E – Platelets

Platelets are involved in blood coagulation. A raised platelet count can occur in infection and malignancy in addition to bleeding. A fall in platelets is seen in bone marrow failure and immune thrombocytopenic purpura.

2. D – Normal red cells

Normal red blood cells lose their nucleus during maturation, giving them their classical bi-concave shape, which provides a high surface area for oxygen carriage.

3. D – Normal red cells

Reticulocytes are the precursor cells for erythrocytes. After being released from the bone marrow into the circulation, they take around a day to fully mature. Reticulocytes normally make up approximately 1% of circulating red cells.

4. C – Megaloblastic cells

Folate deficiency results in the formation of macrocytic megaloblastic cells – large, immature dysfunctional red blood cells.

5. F – Plasma cells

B lymphocytes differentiate into plasma cells. It is these plasma cells that go on to produce antibodies.

ANSWER QUESTION 19

1. E – Factor XIIa

The intrinsic pathway (also known as the contact activation pathway) involves factors VIII, IX, XI and XII.

2. K – Tissue thromboplastin

Tissue thromboplastin (or 'tissue factor') is released during tissue damage and leads to activation of the extrinsic pathway (also known as the tissue factor pathway).

3. C – Factor X

Factor X is activated by factor VIII in the intrinsic pathway and factor VII in the extrinsic pathway.

4. F – Factor XIIIa

Thrombin (factor II) converts fibrinogen (factor I) into a loose fibrin matrix. Activated factor XIII (XIIIa) and calcium subsequently act on this loose fibrin matrix to form a tight fibrin clot.

5. J – Thrombin

Thrombin in the final common pathway of the coagulation cascade activates factor XIII, which stabilizes the fibrin clot.

ANSWER QUESTION 20

1. A – PT: ↑   APTT: ↑   TT: ↔/↑   Platelets: ↓

In liver disease there is decreased production of clotting factors and platelets. There is an increase in PT and APTT. PT tests the extrinsic and common pathways. APTT tests the intrinsic and common pathways.

2. E – PT: ↑   APTT↑   TT: ↑   Platelets: ↔

Heparin inactivates thrombin and factor X, thereby leading to a prolonged APTT and PT, which tests the intrinsic and common pathways and extrinsic and common pathways, respectively. Platelet concentration is normally unaffected except in the case of heparin-induced thrombocytopaenia, where the formation of aberrant antibodies activates platelets with resulting thrombosis.

3. B – PT: ↑   APTT: ↑   TT: ↑   Platelets: ↓

Massive transfusion can lead to a consumptive pathological phenomenon known as disseminated intravascular coagulation (DIC). In DIC there is platelet consumption and reduced clotting leading to prolonged bleeding time and as a result, prolonged APTT and PT.

4. D – PT: ↑   APTT: ↑   TT: ↔   Platelets: ↔

Vitamin K is required for the carboxylation of the factors II, VII, IX and X in the liver. A deficiency in vitamin K therefore impairs the production of these factors and prolongs both the PT and APTT.

5. B – PT: ↑   APTT: ↑   TT: ↑   Platelets: ↓

In DIC there is platelet consumption and clotting factor consumption, which leads to increased bleeding times and prolongation of the PT and APTT.

EMQs Paper 2

1. GASTROENTEROLOGY

A. Common hepatic artery
B. Gastroduodenal artery
C. Left gastric artery
D. Left gastroepiploic artery
E. Right gastric artery
F. Right gastroepiploic artery
G. Short gastric artery
H. None of the above

For each of the following descriptions, select the most appropriate artery. Each option may be used once, more than once or not at all.

1. This artery runs between the layers of the gastrosplenic ligament to reach the fundus of the stomach.
2. This artery is a branch of the gastroduodenal artery.
3. This artery is a small branch of the coeliac trunk.
4. This artery runs between the layers of the greater omentum.
5. This artery runs along the hepatosplenic ligament.

2. GASTROENTEROLOGY

A. Ascending colon
B. Descending colon
C. Duodenum
D. Ileum
E. Jejunum
F. Rectum
G. Transverse colon
H. None of the above

For each of the following descriptions, select the most appropriate part of the gastrointestinal tract. Each option may be used once, more than once or not at all.

1. This is where Peyer patches are classically found.
2. This is where Brunner glands are classically found.
3. This is where Meckel diverticula are classically found.
4. This is where the valvulae conniventes are classically largest.
5. This is where the taeniae coli unite.

25

3. GASTROENTEROLOGY

A. Ileocolic artery
B. Inferior left colic artery
C. Inferior rectal artery
D. Middle colic artery
E. Middle rectal artery
F. Superior left colic artery
G. Superior rectal artery
H. None of the above

For each of the following descriptions, select the most appropriate artery. Each option may be used once, more than once or not at all.

1. This artery supplies the same area as the right colic artery.
2. This is a colic branch of the superior mesenteric artery along with the ileocolic artery and right colic artery.
3. This is a colic branch of the inferior mesenteric artery along with the inferior left colic artery.
4. This artery supplies the descending and sigmoid colon.
5. This artery gives rise to the appendicular artery.

4. GASTROENTEROLOGY

A. Achalasia
B. Adenocarcinoma
C. Barrett oesophagus
D. Duodenal ulcer
E. Gastric ulcer
F. Mallory–Weiss tear
G. Zollinger–Ellison syndrome
H. None of the above

For each of the following scenarios, select the most appropriate diagnosis. Each option may be used once, more than once or not at all.

1. A patient presents with haematemesis. Urgent endoscopy reveals multiple gastric erosions. She is known to be taking omeprazole.
2. A patient presents with weight loss and postprandial epigastric pain. An endoscopic biopsy reveals overexpression of transforming growth factor alpha (TGF-α).
3. A patient presents with recurrent regurgitation of fluids and solids. A barium meal reveals a beak-like tapering in the lower oesophagus.
4. A patient presents with haematemesis after drinking 12 pints of lager.
5. An elderly patient presents with a recent history of weight loss and anorexia. Endoscopy reveals a thickened, stiff gastric wall.

5. GASTROENTEROLOGY

A. *Bacillus cereus*
B. *Giardia lamblia*
C. *Helicobacter pylori*
D. *Listeria monocytogenes*
E. Rotavirus
F. *Salmonella typhi*
G. *Staphylococcus aureus*
H. None of the above

For each of the following descriptions, select the most appropriate organism. Each option may be used once, more than once or not at all.

1. A patient presents with severe nausea, vomiting and diarrhoea approximately 8 hours after eating a poorly reheated Chinese takeaway meal.
2. This organism is only transmitted by humans and multiplies in Peyer patches. Resulting infection has a slow onset and has pathognomonic Rose spots.
3. This organism causes foul smelling non-bloody diarrhoea. The organism parasite contains two nuclei, each with four flagella and a ventral adhesive disc.
4. This organism causes extremely watery diarrhoea through the stimulation of the enteric nervous system with enterotoxins.
5. This organism is almost always found in patients with duodenal ulceration.

6. LYMPHATIC SYSTEM

A. Axillary lymph nodes
B. Cisterna chyli
C. Deep inguinal lymph nodes
D. Left brachiocephalic artery
E. Left subclavian vein
F. Para-aortic lymph nodes
G. Pre-aortic lymph nodes
H. Right brachiocephalic artery
I. Right internal jugular vein
J. Thoracic duct

For each of the following descriptions, select the most appropriate lymph node group or vessel type. Each option may be used once, more than once or not at all.

1. The site of drainage of the right lymphatic duct.
2. The site of drainage of lymph from the testes.
3. A common drainage area for lymph from the entire lower limb and abdomen.

4. The site of drainage of the thoracic duct.
5. A common drainage area for most of the body's lymph which itself drains indirectly into the heart.

7. LYMPHATIC SYSTEM

A. Cortex
B. Cuboidal epithelium
C. Fibrous capsule
D. Follicular layer
E. Immune network
F. Medulla
G. Paracortex
H. Reticular network
 I. Subcapsular sinus

For each of the following descriptions, select the most appropriate region of the lymph node. Each option may be used once, more than once or not at all.

1. The outer layer of a lymph node.
2. The network of fixed macrophages, interdigitating dendritic cells and lymphocytes embedded in lymphatic channels.
3. The region of the lymph node predominantly containing antibody-secreting plasma cells.
4. The region of the lymph node containing B-cells, macrophages and dendritic cells organized into primary follicles.
5. The region of the lymph node containing predominantly T-cells and interdigitating dendritic cells.

8. NEPHROLOGY

A. Bowman's capsule
B. Collecting duct
C. Distal convoluted tubule
D. Loop of Henle: descending limb
E. Loop of Henle: thick ascending limb
F. Proximal tubule
G. Renal artery
H. Renal cortex
 I. Renal medulla
J. Vasa recta

For each of the following statements, select the correct anatomical location. Each option may be used once, more than once or not at all.

1. The location of the majority of HCO_3^- reabsorption.
2. Antidiuretic hormone acts by binding to V2 vasopressin receptors at this location.

3. The site of the $Na^+/K^+/Cl^-$ cotransporter.
4. The site of glomerular filtration.
5. A site which is only permeable to water and does not transport solute.

9. URINARY SYSTEM

A. 20.8 mL/min
B. 24.6 mL/min
C. 25.9 mL/min
D. 65.7 mL/min
E. 73.4 mL/min
F. 74.3 mL/min
G. 77.9 mL/min
H. 89.9 mL/min
I. 125.0 mL/min
J. 184.5 mL/min

For each of the following scenarios, calculate the estimated creatinine clearance, using the Cockcroft–Gault formula, provided below. Each option may be used once, more than once or not at all.

$$\text{Creatinine clearance} = \frac{(140 - \text{Age}) \times \text{Weight} \times K}{\text{Serum creatinine}}$$

The constant term K is 1.23 for males and 1.04 for females.

1. An 80-year-old man weighing 60 kg has a urea of 24 mmol/L and creatinine of 180 µmol/L.
2. A 20-year-old girl presents with loin pain and haematuria. Her urea and electrolytes show a urea of 12 mmol/L and creatinine of 95 µmol/L and her weight is 50 kg.
3. A 35-year-old pregnant woman weighs 70 kg. Her blood pressure is 139/80 mmHg and bedside tests show ++ glucose in her urine. Her urea is 7 mmol/L and creatinine is 85 µmol/L.
4. A 60-year-old man with suspected malignancy weighs 50 kg. His creatinine is 190 µmol/L.
5. A 40-year-old woman who is due to be prescribed a low molecular weight heparin has a serum creatinine of 85 µmol/L. Her most recent weight, measured 2 weeks ago, was 60 kg.

10. URINARY SYSTEM

A. Aldosterone
B. Blood glucose
C. Blood pressure
D. Decrease
E. Follicle stimulating hormone
F. Glucose

G. Human chorionic gonadotrophin
H. Increase
 I. Luteinizing hormone
 J. No change
K. Progesterone
 L. Protein

For each of the following, select the most appropriate answer. Each option may be used once, more than once or not at all.

1. Which substance is tested for in the urine if pregnancy is suspected?
2. This urinary solute helps detect gestational diabetes.
3. How does pregnancy affect the glomerular filtration rate?
4. Which substance in the urine may suggest pre-eclampsia?
5. Which parameter, other than that of the previous answer, is elevated in pre-eclampsia?

11. NEUROLOGY

A. Arachnoid villi
B. Cerebral aqueduct of Sylvius
C. Foramen of Luschka
D. Foramina of Monro
E. Fourth ventricle
 F. Lateral ventricles
G. Subarachnoid space
H. Third ventricle

For each of the following descriptions, select the most appropriate part of the brain. Each option may be used once, more than once or not at all.

1. This is located in the cleft between the two thalami.
2. This connects the lateral ventricles to the third ventricle.
3. These are separated from each other by the septum pellucidum.
4. This connects the third and fourth ventricle.
5. The roof of this structure is formed by the cerebellum.

12. NEUROLOGY

A. Anterior cerebral artery
B. Anterior choroidal artery
C. Anterior communicating artery
D. Internal carotid artery
E. Middle cerebral artery
 F. Middle meningeal artery
G. Posterior cerebral artery
H. Posterior communicating artery

For each of the following descriptions, select the most appropriate arteries. Each option may be used once, more than once or not at all.

1. The terminal branch of the internal carotid artery which does not take part in the circle of Willis.
2. The communication between the anterior circulation and the posterior cerebral artery.
3. The communication between the left and right anterior cerebral arteries.
4. The third part of the first branch of the maxillary artery.
5. This artery supplies the choroid plexus of the lateral and third ventricles.

13. NEUROLOGY

A. CN III
B. CN VI
C. CN VII
D. CN VIII
E. CN IX
F. CN X
G. CN XI
H. CN XII

For each of the following descriptions, select the most appropriate cranial nerve. Each option may be used once, more than once or not at all.

1. This cranial nerve supplies motor fibres to the stapedius.
2. This cranial nerve contains preganglionic parasympathetic fibres with cell bodies in the Edinger–Westphal nucleus.
3. This cranial nerve innervates hair cells of the cochlear.
4. This cranial nerve enters the skull through the foramen magnum to leave through the jugular foramen.
5. This cranial nerve provides branches to the carotid sinus.

14. NEUROLOGY

A. Left accessory nerve
B. Left hypoglossal nerve
C. Left trigeminal nerve
D. Left vagus nerve
E. Lower motor neuron facial nerve
F. Right accessory nerve
G. Right glossopharyngeal nerve
H. Right hypoglossal nerve
 I. Right trigeminal nerve
 J. Right vagus nerve
K. Upper motor neuron facial nerve

For each of the following, select the most appropriate nerve, damage to which would result in the given examination finding. Each option may be used once, more than once or not at all.

1. Drooping of the left side of the face without sparing of the forehead
2. Tongue deviation to the left
3. Jaw deviation to the right
4. Uvula deviation to the right
5. Drooping of the left shoulder

15. NEUROLOGY

A. Anterior cerebral artery
B. Anterior communicating artery
C. Circle of Willis
D. Left middle cerebral artery
E. Left posterior cerebral artery
F. Posterior cerebral arteries
G. Right middle cerebral artery
H. Right posterior cerebral artery

For each of the following scenarios, select the most appropriate site of the cerebrovascular lesion. Each option may be used once, more than once or not at all.

1. An 82-year-old woman presents to accident and emergency having developed sudden-onset sensory and motor loss on the right with slurring of speech.
2. A 67-year-old man presents with sudden-onset loss of vision in the left eye.
3. A 45-year-old bus driver presents with sudden-onset headache and loss of consciousness.
4. After a 67-year-old patient recovered from a stroke, relatives have noticed a change in personality and behaviour.
5. A 72-year-old patient is adamant that he is not blind but walks into the furniture.

16. NEUROLOGY

A. Acromegaly
B. Addison disease
C. Cushing syndrome
D. Hypopituitarism
E. Hypothyroidism
F. Pseudohypoparathyroidism
G. Syndrome of inappropriate antidiuretic hormone secretion (SIADH)
H. Thyrotoxicosis

For each of the following descriptions, select the most appropriate diagnosis. Each option may be used once, more than once or not at all.

1. This condition is associated with onycholysis and pretibial myxoedema.
2. This condition is associated with hair loss and pale skin.
3. This condition is associated with macrognathia and coarse facial features.
4. This condition is associated with tinged, thin skin and looking older than one's actual age.
5. This condition is associated with abdominal striae and supraclavicular fat pads.

17. ENDOCRINOLOGY

A. Addison disease
B. Cushing disease
C. Hyperthyroidism
D. Hypothyroidism
E. Sick euthyroidism
F. Subclinical hyperthyroidism
G. Subclinical hypothyroidism
H. Thyroid hormone resistance

For each of the following blood test results, select the most appropriate condition. Each option may be used once, more than once or not at all.

1. High TSH and low T4
2. Low TSH and high T4
3. Low TSH, T4 and T3
4. High TSH and high T4
5. Low TSH and normal T4

18. ENDOCRINOLOGY

A. Adrenalectomy
B. Immediate cessation of steroid treatment
C. Metyrapone
D. Pituitary radiotherapy
E. Transcranial approach
F. Trans-pharyngeal approach
G. Trans-sphenoidal approach
H. Weaning course of steroids

For each of the following descriptions, select the most appropriate method. Each option may be used once, more than once or not at all.

1. This is the treatment of iatrogenic Cushing syndrome.
2. This approach is used in treatment of Cushing disease.
3. This may be done post-adrenalectomy to prevent Nelson syndrome.

4. This is performed to treat adrenal carcinoma.
5. This may be used in the initial treatment of Cushing disease.

19. ENDOCRINOLOGY

A. At midnight
B. Bilateral temporal hemianopia
C. Bilateral temporal quadrantanopia
D. In the early morning
E. Pseudo-Cushing syndrome
F. The hypothalamus and pituitary
G. The hypothalamus only
H. The pituitary only
 I. Unilateral temporal hemianopia
 J. Urinary free cortisol

For each of the following descriptions, select the most appropriate option. Each option may be used once, more than once or not at all.

1. The visual defect resulting from a large pituitary adenoma.
2. In a patient who drinks excess alcohol but has clinical symptoms and signs for Cushing syndrome, the initial investigation in this condition may be falsely positive.
3. Cortisol is highest at this time of the day.
4. Cortisol can be excreted from the body in this form.
5. Negative feedback from cortisol affects this/these area(s).

20. ENDOCRINOLOGY

A. Adrenal metastases
B. Autoimmune disease
C. Congenital
D. Hyperpigmentation of palmar creases and buccal mucosa, and postural hypotension
E. Hypertension, bradycardia and a reduced consciousness
F. Hypotension, tachycardia and a reduced consciousness
G. Tuberculosis
H. Weakness, weight loss, dizziness and fatigue

For each of the following descriptions, select the most appropriate response. Each option may be used once, more than once or not at all.

1. This is the most common cause of Addison disease worldwide.
2. This is the most common cause of Addison disease in the UK.
3. These are the typical signs of Addison disease.
4. These are the typical signs of an Addisonian crisis.
5. These are the typical symptoms of Addison disease.

Answers Paper 2

ANSWER QUESTION 1

1. G – Short gastric artery
2. F – Right gastroepiploic artery
3. C – Left gastric artery
4. D – Left gastroepiploic artery
5. C – Left gastric artery

The stomach is supplied by all three branches of the coeliac trunk. The left gastric artery is a small branch of the trunk and runs between the layers of the lesser omentum or the hepatosplenic ligament. It supplies both surfaces of the stomach. The right gastric artery is a branch of the common hepatic artery. The left gastroepiploic artery is a branch of the splenic artery. It runs along the greater curvature of the stomach through the layer of the greater omentum. The right gastroepiploic is a branch of the gastroduodenal artery and supplies the right side of the stomach and the superior part of the duodenum. The short gastric arteries are also a branch of the splenic artery. They run between the layers of the gastro-splenic ligament to supply the fundus of the stomach.

ANSWER QUESTION 2

1. D – Ileum
2. C – Duodenum
3. D – Ileum
4. E – Jejunum
5. F – Rectum

Peyer patches are generally found in the ileum and Brunner glands are typically found in the duodenum, although they can be found in other places throughout the gastrointestinal tract. Meckel diverticula are classically found in the ileum as a persistence of the embryonic vitel-line (omphalomesenteric) duct. They affect 2% of the population, are usually located 2 feet from the ileocaecal valve, are 2 inches in length and involve two types of ectopic tissue (gastric and pancreatic). Patients often present at 2 years of age and males are twice as likely to be affected. Valvulae conniventes (also known as circular folds, plicae circulares or valves of Kerckring) are largest in the proximal half of the jejunum.

Taeniae coli – the three longitudinal bands of smooth muscle on the outside of the colon – converge at the appendix and fan out to unite at the rectosigmoid junction.

ANSWER QUESTION 3

1. A – Ileocolic artery
2. D – Middle colic artery
3. F – Superior left colic artery
4. G – Superior rectal artery
5. A – Ileocolic artery

The blood supply of the colon is supplied as follows: the ascending colon is supplied by the ileocolic and right colic arteries; the proximal transverse colon is supplied by the middle colic artery; the distal transverse colon is supplied by the superior left colic artery; and the descending and sigmoid colon is supplied by the inferior left colic artery. The appendicular artery is a terminal branch of the ileocolic artery. The branches of the superior mesenteric artery are the inferior pancreaticoduodenal artery (supplies the pancreatic head and inferior duodenum), intestinal arteries (give branches to the ileum and jejunum), and the ileocolic, right colic and middle colic arteries. The branches of the inferior mesenteric artery are the left colic artery, sigmoid arteries (between two and four), and the superior rectal artery (the terminal branch).

ANSWER QUESTION 4

1. G – Zollinger–Ellison syndrome
2. H – None of the above
3. A – Achalasia
4. F – Mallory–Weiss tear
5. B – Adenocarcinoma

Zollinger–Ellison syndrome is a rare condition where there is an abnormal increase in gastrin leading to an increase in HCl acid in the stomach, which results in severe ulceration. (Note that it may be linked to multiple endocrine neoplasia type 1 [MEN 1] syndrome, in which patients also have pituitary and parathyroid tumours in up to 25% of cases.) Ménétrier disease is also known as hyperplastic hypersecretory gastropathy. This is a condition where the patient has an overexpression of TGF-α leading to hypertrophy of the gastric mucosal folds. The patient then oversecretes mucus, lowering plasma protein levels. Achalasia is the abnormal failure of relaxation of the lower oesophageal sphincter. On barium swallow a typical bird's beak pattern is shown. A stiff, thickened 'leather bottle stomach' (linitis plastica) is seen in diffuse stomach adenocarcinoma. This appearance can be seen on both direct endoscopy and a barium meal.

ANSWER QUESTION 5

1. A – *Bacillus cereus*
2. F – *Salmonella typhi*
3. B – *Giardia lamblia*
4. E – Rotavirus
5. C – *Helicobacter pylori*

Bacillus cereus is responsible for severe nausea, vomiting and diarrhoea. The emetic form is commonly caused by eating undercooked rice. The *Salmonella typhi* Rose spots are bacterial emboli in the skin and occur in up to one-third of patients. Rotavirus is a double-stranded RNA, 'wheel-like' virus which replicates in the mucosa of the small intestine to cause secretory diarrhoea with no inflammation. *Helicobacter pylori* is a Gram-negative bacterium found in up to 90% of patients with duodenal ulceration and up to 70% of those with gastric ulceration.

ANSWER QUESTION 6

1. I – Right internal jugular vein
The right lymphatic duct drains the right deep cervical, axillary and bronchomediastinal lymph node groups. It then drains into the right internal jugular vein or the right subclavian vein.

2. F – Para-aortic lymph nodes
A common misconception is that testicular lymphatic drainage is to the inguinal nodes, but this is not correct, as the embryological origin of the testes is from the abdomen. They descend into the scrotum in foetal life from the abdomen. Their blood and lymphatic supply is therefore derived from the abdomen. This is clinically important, as testicular cancer will therefore not present with inguinal lymphadenopathy unless there has been spread of tumour cells into the scrotal skin.

3. B – Cisterna chyli
The cisterna chyli is a collecting vessel which drains the pre-aortic, para-aortic and deep inguinal nodes from both the left and right sides. Lymph from it drains into the thoracic duct and thence into the right atrium.

4. E – Left subclavian vein
All lymph in the body, except for that draining from the right deep cervical, axillary and bronchomediastinal lymph node groups into the right lymphatic duct, drains into the heart via the thoracic duct and left subclavian vein.

5. J – Thoracic duct
The thoracic duct drains lymph from the cisterna chyli (which drains lymph from the entire lower limbs and abdomen), the left deep cervical nodes, left axillary nodes and left bronchomediastinal nodes. It drains

into the left suclavian vein, which itself drains into the superior vena cava via the brachiocephalic vein, and then into the right atrium of the heart.

ANSWER QUESTION 7

1. C – Fibrous capsule

Mucosal-associated lymphoid tissue (MALT) is much more loosely organized, arranged either as collections of lymphocytes and macrophages or primary lymphoid follicles, and thus MALT are not encapsulated in contrast to lymph nodes.

2. H – Reticular network

Reticular macrophages directly phagocytose antibody-tagged bacteria.

3. F – Medulla

The medulla is more sparsely populated with lymphocytes than the lymph node cortex and paracortex.

4. A – Cortex

The cortex is the main B-cell area of the lymph node and cells are arranged into primary follicles, which enlarge on antigen exposure to become secondary follicles. The cortex is also known as the thymus-independent area.

5. G – Paracortex

The paracortex is also known as the thymus-dependent area. Interdigitating dendritic cells are involved in antigen presentation to the T-cells within this region through major histocompatibility complex class II molecules.

ANSWER QUESTION 8

1. F – Proximal tubule

The proximal tubule is the site at which the majority (approximately two-thirds) of filtered solutes and water are reabsorbed. Reabsorption at the proximal tubule is isotonic and reabsorption of solutes is dependent on epithelial sodium transport mechanisms (e.g. the sodium–glucose transporter [SGLT] and sodium–hydrogen exchange [NHE]).

2. B – Collecting duct

Antidiuretic hormone (ADH) is secreted by the posterior pituitary in response to increased plasma osmolarity, as detected by osmoreceptors of the hypothalamus. It acts to reduce the elevated osmolarity by conserving water. To do so, ADH binds to V2 vasopressin receptors on the basolateral membrane of the collecting duct, which results in the insertion of aquaporin II channels into the apical membrane. This increases the permeability of the collecting duct to water, and the hyperosmotic interstitium facilitates water conservation.

3. E – Loop of Henle: thick ascending limb

The $Na^+/K^+/Cl^-$ cotransporter (NKCC) facilitates the active transport of sodium, potassium and chloride at the thick ascending limb of the loop of Henle. The loop diuretics (e.g. furosemide) act on NKCCs. They inhibit chloride reabsorption and cause natriuresis. Because water follows sodium, diuresis ensues. Inhibition of the NKCC means that potassium ions are also excreted, which can lead to hypokalaemia if sufficient potassium supplementation is not given.

4. A – Bowman's capsule

Bowman's capsule surrounds the glomerulus and is the site of filtration. The filtration barrier is made up of the capillary cell wall, podocytes and the fused basement membrane. The net filtration pressure is dependent on the hydrostatic and colloid osmotic forces across the glomerular capillaries. The composition of the glomerular filtrate is identical to plasma, except for the absence of proteins, which are too large to pass through the filtration barrier.

5. D – Loop of Henle: descending limb

The descending limb of the loop of Henle is permeable only to water and does not facilitate the transport of solutes. It is made up of thin, flattened squamous epithelium with few mitochondria, because there is limited active transport. The nephron is specialized in this way to allow the generation of urine with an appropriate composition for osmotic homeostasis and to retain essential solutes.

ANSWER QUESTION 9

1. B – 24.6 mL/min

Estimating creatinine clearance with the Cockcroft–Gault formula is a useful measurement of renal function. An estimated creatinine clearance or glomerular filtration rate (GFR) is vital when prescribing potentially nephrotoxic drugs. Poor renal function can result in higher levels of drugs and toxins in the blood, as the kidneys are unable to effectively excrete it. (See the British National Formulary for details of safe prescribing in renal impairment.)

$$\text{Estimated creatinine clearance} = \frac{(140-80)\times 60\times 1.23}{180} = 24.6\,\text{mL/min}$$

2. D – 65.7 mL/min

$$\text{Estimated creatinine clearance} = \frac{(140-20)\times 50\times 1.04}{95} = 65.7\,\text{mL/min}$$

Renal calculi classically present with severe colicky 'loin to groin' pain and may be associated with nausea and vomiting. Haematuria may also be a feature, as in this scenario. If there are no signs of obstruction, management is conservative and includes increasing fluid intake and analgesia (e.g. diclofenac).

3. H – 89.9 mL/min

$$\text{Estimated creatinine clearance} = \frac{(140-35)\times70\times1.04}{85} = 89.9\,\text{mL/min}$$

Blood pressure and urinary glucose and protein are monitored carefully in pregnant women. High urinary protein in the presence of hypertension may indicate pre-eclampsia. Pre-eclampsia occurs after 20 weeks' gestation and resolves following the birth of the foetus. Hypertension should be managed carefully in an attempt to prevent eclampsia, which is a major cause of maternal mortality.

4. C – 25.9 mL/min

$$\text{Estimated creatinine clearance} = \frac{(140-60)\times50\times1.23}{190} = 25.9\,\text{mL/min}$$

Carcinoma of the bladder classically presents with painless haematuria. It is associated with a history of smoking and work in the dye industry. Most tumours are of transitional cell origin, although squamous cell carcinoma occurs in 2% and is associated with schistosomiasis.

5. E – 73.4 mL/min

$$\text{Estimated creatinine clearance} = \frac{(140-40)\times60\times1.04}{85} = 73.4\,\text{mL/min}$$

It is important to estimate creatinine clearance before prescribing medications to patients. All hospital patients should be given daily subcutaneous lower molecular weight heparin (e.g. clexane) to prevent thromboembolic disease. If creatinine clearance is low (e.g. <60 mL/min) this dose should be halved to 20 mg.

ANSWER QUESTION 10

1. G – Human chorionic gonadotrophin
Urinary pregnancy tests use urinary levels of human chorionic gonadotrophin (hCG) to detect whether implantation has occurred. Blood tests are more sensitive at detecting pregnancy, but urinary tests can be bought over the counter and performed at home. Home ovulation kits have also been developed in order to improve the chances of conceiving. They detect urinary luteinizing hormone (LH). The LH surge precedes ovulation by about 36 hours, at which point the woman is most likely to conceive. The blood test used to detect ovulation is usually the day 21 progesterone, which is used to check that ovulation is occurring, for example in a woman with subfertility.

2. F – Glucose
Glycosuria is found on routine urine dipstick tests in gestational diabetes. The diagnosis is confirmed with a blood glucose level (fasting, 2 hours post-glucose load, or random). It is thought that the change in hormonal concentrations may lead to a relative insulin deficiency in the second or third trimester of pregnancy, which results in gestational diabetes. Most cases resolve after delivery but the mother is at a higher risk of developing diabetes mellitus later on in life. Babies of diabetic mothers are more likely to be large for gestational age (macrosomia) and have hypoglycaemia.

3. H – Increase
Glomerular filtration rate (GFR) increases by about 40% in pregnancy as renal blood flow increases to meet the additional demands. GFR is a measure of renal function and is determined by the hydrostatic and osmotic forces across the glomerular capillaries, arterial pressure and vascular resistance.

4. L – Protein
Pre-eclampsia, or pregnancy-induced hypertension, is carefully monitored at antenatal visits. It develops from about the 20th week of gestation and is associated with high levels of proteinuria. Peripheral and facial oedemas commonly coexist. It is most common in primigravid women and in those who suffer with hypertension, diabetes and autoimmune disorders. Pre-eclampsia can progress to the life-threatening condition of eclampsia, which is characterized by convulsions. Magnesium sulphate can be used to prevent seizures.

5. C – Blood pressure
Hypertension and proteinuria occur with pre-eclampsia. Headaches, visual disturbance and convulsions occur in eclampsia. Mothers with pre-eclampsia are also at higher risk of HELLP syndrome (haemolysis, elevated liver enzymes and low platelets). Babies of pre-eclamptic mothers are commonly small for gestational age, probably owing to placental insufficiency.

ANSWER QUESTION 11

1. H – Third ventricle
The third ventricle lies in a cleft between the two thalami. It communicates anteriorly with the lateral ventricles via the foramina of Monro and posteroinferiorly with the fourth ventricle via the cerebral aqueduct.

2. D – Foramina of Monro
The right and left foramina of Monro (or interventricular foramen) connect the lateral ventricles to the third ventricle.

3. F – Lateral ventricles

The two lateral ventricles are separated from each other by a median partition, the septum pellucidum.

4. B – Cerebral aqueduct of Sylvius

The cerebral aqueduct of Sylvius connects the third and fourth ventricles.

5. E – Fourth ventricle

The fourth ventricle is located in the hindbrain. Its roof is formed by the ventral surface of the cerebellum. Its floor is formed by the rhomboid fossa and its lateral walls by the cerebellar peduncles.

ANSWER QUESTION 12

1. E – Middle cerebral artery

The middle cerebral artery is a terminal branch of the internal carotid artery. It does not take part in the circle of Willis. The middle cerebral artery comprises four parts: M1, also known as the sphenoidal segment; M2, also known as the insular segment; M3, also known as the opercular segment; and M4, also known as the terminal segment.

2. H – Posterior communicating artery

The posterior communicating artery communicates anteriorly with the trifurcation of the internal carotid artery and posteriorly with the posterior cerebral artery.

3. C – Anterior communicating artery

The anterior communicating artery unites the left and right anterior cerebral arteries.

4. F – Middle meningeal artery

The middle meningeal artery is the third branch of the first part of the maxillary artery. It supplies and runs between the dura, and damage can result in an extradural haemorrhage.

5. B – Anterior choroidal artery

The anterior choroidal artery usually arises from the internal carotid artery. It supplies the choroid plexus of the ventricles as well as the limbic structures and basal ganglia.

ANSWER QUESTION 13

1. C – CN VII

The facial nerve (CN VII) gives rise to the stapedial nerve which supplies motor fibres to the stapedius.

2. A – CN III

The oculomotor nerve (CN III) enters the orbit through the superior orbital fissure. It contains parasympathetic fibres which mediate the efferent limb of the pupillary light reflex. The preganglionic fibres originate in the Edinger–Westphal nucleus. The postganglionic fibres lie in the ciliary ganglion.

3. D – CN VIII

The vestibulocochlear nerve (CN VIII) has both cochlear and vestibular fibres. It innervates the hair cells of the cochlea (organ of Corti) and mediates hearing/equilibrium.

4. G – CN XI

The accessory nerve (CN XI) has a small cranial root and a larger spinal root. Its spinal root arises from the upper five segments of the spinal cord and passes superiorly to enter the skull through the foramen magnum. It leaves the skull through the jugular foramen.

5. E – CN IX

The glossopharyngeal nerve (CN IX) gives rise to a carotid sinus branch. This supplies afferent fibres to the carotid sinus and carotid body. It mediates the afferent component of the carotid sinus/body reflex.

ANSWER QUESTION 14

1. E – Lower motor neuron facial nerve

This patient presents with features of Bell's palsy. This is a lower motor neuron lesion of the facial nerve (CN VII). In a lesion of the upper motor neuron, there is usually sparing of the forehead because of contralateral innervation.

2. B – Left hypoglossal nerve

This is a lesion of the left hypoglossal nerve (CN XII). The tongue deviates towards the side of the lesion.

3. I – Right trigeminal nerve

This is a lesion of the right trigeminal nerve (CN V). The jaw deviates towards the side of the lesion.

4. D – Left vagus nerve

This is a lesion in the left vagus nerve (CN X). The uvula deviates away from the side of the lesion.

5. A – Left accessory nerve

This is a lesion of the left accessory nerve (CN XI). The shoulder droops on the side of the lesion (trapezius weakness). There is also weakness turning the head to the contralateral side of the lesion (sternocleidomastoid weakness).

ANSWER QUESTION 15

1. D – Left middle cerebral artery

The middle cerebral artery is a terminal branch of the internal carotid artery. It supplies the sensory and motor areas around the central sulcus as well as the auditory and language centres. The symptoms on the right indicate the lesion is in the left artery. Note that the left (dominant) hemisphere is the site of the language centres.

2. H – Right posterior cerebral artery
The posterior cerebral artery is a terminal branch of the basilar artery. It supplies the cortex and white matter of the occipital lobe. Lesions in the posterior cerebral artery produce a contralateral homonymous hemianopia. There is often macular sparing because of the collateral supply via the middle cerebral artery.

3. C – Circle of Willis
This patient presents with symptoms of a subarachnoid haemorrhage. The most common causes of subarachnoid haemorrhage are cerebral aneurysms. They are most commonly found in the circle of Willis.

4. A – Anterior cerebral artery
The anterior cerebral artery is a terminal branch of the internal carotid artery. It supplies the frontal lobe, which is associated with behaviour and personality.

5. F – Posterior cerebral arteries
This patient has Anton syndrome – also known as visual anosognosia. Affected people are blind but are adamant that they can actually see. It is associated with bilateral occipital strokes.

ANSWER QUESTION 16

1. H – Thyrotoxicosis
High free levels of T4 and a suppressed thyroid-stimulating hormone (TSH) would give rise to hyperthyroidism and thyrotoxicosis. Other features include irritability, anxiety, palpitations, feeling hot and sweaty, weight loss, atrial fibrillation, hair loss, exophthalmos and ophthalmoplegia.

2. E – Hypothyroidism
Low levels of T4 and a high TSH would give rise to hypothyroidism. Other features include feeling cold, weight gain and depression.

3. A – Acromegaly
Acromegaly occurs secondary to high levels of growth hormone secretion from the anterior pituitary. Cardiovascular and gastroenterological risks are associated with the disease. Most patients require colonoscopy at the age of 50 to look for malignancy. The disease is also associated with impaired glucose tolerance.

4. D – Hypopituitarism
Hypopituitarism can lead to tinged, thin skin and facial wrinkling, making the patient appear older.

5. C – Cushing syndrome

Cushing syndrome is due to prolonged high levels of cortisol. Other features include high blood pressure, central obesity, thin skin, proximal muscle weakness and irregular menstruation. Causes of Cushing syndrome include long-term steroid use and a benign ACTH-secreting pituitary adenoma (Cushing disease).

ANSWER QUESTION 17

1. D – Hypothyroidism

Hypothyroidism results in low levels of T4 and high TSH.

2. C – Hyperthyroidism

Hyperthyroidism is associated with high levels of T4 and low TSH.

3. E – Sick euthyroidism

During times of systemic illness, the circulating levels of all the thyroid hormones tend to be low. These need to be rechecked once the patient has recovered.

4. H – Thyroid hormone resistance

High TSH and high T4 can be due to either thyroid hormone resistance or a TSH secreting tumour.

5. F – Subclinical hyperthyroidism

Subclinical hyperthyroidism can be monitored by the GP. If there are associated clinical signs, then the patient may benefit from treatment, and the risks and benefits of this must be evaluated.

ANSWER QUESTION 18

1. H – Weaning course of steroids

Depending on the disease, physicians should try to wean patients from steroids while avoiding immediate relapse of underlying disease.

2. G – Trans-sphenoidal approach

A trans-sphenoidal approach for the surgical removal of pituitary adenomas is usually appropriate.

3. D – Pituitary radiotherapy

Adrenalectomy leads to abolition of negative feedback and overproduction of ACTH. This can lead to Nelson syndrome. Radiotherapy to the pituitary may prevent this.

4. A – Adrenalectomy

Adrenalectomy alone rarely manages to successfully treat adrenal carcinoma, and adjuvant chemoradiotherapy is usually required. Adrenalectomy is effective in benign adenomas.

5. C – Metyrapone

Metyrapone and ketoconazole may be prescribed prior to surgery in Cushing disease to reduce cortisol secretion.

ANSWER QUESTION 19

1. B – Bilateral temporal hemianopia

Because of the decussation of the optic fibres at the optic chiasm, compression by a pituitary tumour of the optic chiasm leads to loss of vision in both eyes in the temporal visual field (i.e. tunnel vision).

2. E – Pseudo-Cushing syndrome

Pseudo-Cushing syndrome may be present on an overnight dexamethasone suppression test if a patient drinks alcohol to excess, is obese, is depressed or takes any drugs such as rifampicin or phenytoin which lead to an increased dexamethasone metabolism.

3. D – In the early morning

Cortisol is secreted in a diurnal fashion, with the highest levels in the morning. This must be taken into account when performing diagnostic tests such as the dexamethasone suppression test.

4. J – Urinary free cortisol

Cortisol can also be excreted as 17-oxygenic steroids.

5. F – The hypothalamus and pituitary

Cortisol feeds back to the pituitary and hypothalamus to inhibit secretion of adrenocorticotrophic hormone and corticotrophin releasing factor, respectively.

ANSWER QUESTION 20

1. G – Tuberculosis

Worldwide, the most common cause of Addison disease is tuberculosis, which causes destruction of the adrenal gland. Addison disease (or adrenal insufficiency) causes low levels of cortisol (and often aldosterone) to be produced. Cortisol is responsible for maintaining blood pressure and cardiovascular function in addition to its roles in metabolism and glycaemic control.

2. B – Autoimmune disease

In the UK, Addison disease most commonly occurs secondary to autoimmune disease.

3. D – Hyperpigmentation of palmar creases and buccal mucosa, and postural hypotension

Hyperpigmentation is due to increased levels of adrenocorticotrophic hormone, which is cleaved from its precursor proopiomelanocortin (POMC). POMC is also the precursor of melanin, and so high levels cause skin pigmentation.

4. F – Hypotension, tachycardia and a reduced consciousness

An Addisonian crisis may be precipitated by infection, trauma or surgery, when metabolic demand increases. Symptoms of a crisis include sudden abdominal pain, severe vomiting, profound hypotension and loss of consciousness. It can be fatal if not recognized and treated promptly. Treatment includes fluid resuscitation and IV hydrocortisone.

5. H – Weakness, weight loss, dizziness and fatigue

Addison disease can be difficult to diagnose clinically and is often diagnosed late due to the non-specificity of the symptoms/signs. Clues to look out for include hyperpigmentation, hyponatraemia and hyperkalaemia; a past medical history of other autoimmune conditions may suggest a diagnosis of Addison disease.

EMQs Paper 3

1. PHARMACOLOGY

A. Angiotensin-converting enzyme inhibitors
B. Beta-blockers
C. Calcium channel blockers
D. Hydralazine
E. Loop diuretics
F. Methyldopa
G. Minoxidil
H. Potassium-sparing diuretics

For each of the following descriptions, select the most appropriate drug. Each option may be used once, more than once or not at all.

1. This drug is the first-line management option for a 39-year-old Nigerian man with hypertension.
2. A 39-year-old Caucasian man requires initiation of treatment for hypertension. Name the class of drugs most appropriate in this case.
3. A 67-year-old female patient is already on enalapril; however, she requires further antihypertensive medications. She suffers with gout. Name the class of drugs most appropriate in this case.
4. This drug can cause hypertrichosis.
5. This drug can result in nightmares.

2. PHARMACOLOGY

A. Adenosine
B. Amiodarone
C. Bisoprolol
D. Digoxin
E. Flecainide
F. Lidocaine
G. Sotalol
H. Verapamil

For each of the following descriptions, select the most appropriate drug. Each option may be used once, more than once or not at all.

1. This drug must *not* be used in patients with Wolff–Parkinson–White syndrome.

2. Slate-grey skin, corneal microdeposits and pulmonary fibrosis are all associated with this drug.
3. A 66-year-old woman presents with atrial fibrillation at a rate of 120 bpm. She has no other medical problems. This is the first-line option rate control.
4. This drug can cause the feeling of an impending sense of doom, chest tightness, throat tightness and facial flushing when administered.
5. This drug may cause hyperthyroidism.

3. PHARMACOLOGY

A. Amiloride
B. Bendroflumethiazide
C. Doxazosin
D. Enalapril
E. Finasteride
F. Furosemide
G. Losartan
H. Mannitol
I. Spironolactone
J. Tamsulosin

For each of the following adverse effects, select the single most commonly implicated drug. Each option may be used once, more than once or not at all.

1. Dry cough
2. Gynaecomastia
3. Ototoxicity
4. Hyperuricaemia
5. Thrombophlebitis

4. PHARMACOLOGY

A. They affect anticodon recognition, which leads to the misreading of the DNA
B. They affect DNA gyrase
C. They cause premature termination of the peptide chain
D. They compete with tRNA for the A site
E. They have no effect on any of these
F. They inhibit translocation
G. They inhibit transpeptidation

For each of the following descriptions, select the most appropriate mechanisms of action. Each option may be used once, more than once or not at all.

1. Macrolides
2. Sulphonamides

3. Fluoroquinolones
4. Aminoglycosides
5. Beta-lactams

5. PHARMACOLOGY

A. Chemical antagonism
B. Competitive antagonism
C. Equilibrium antagonism
D. Functional antagonism
E. Non-competitive antagonism
F. Pharmacokinetic antagonism
G. Physiological antagonism
H. Reactive antagonism

For each of the following descriptions, select the most appropriate antagonistic reaction. Each option may be used once, more than once or not at all.

1. The antagonist drug reacts with an agonist molecule, rendering it useless.
2. The antagonist drug competes for the same binding site on the receptor as the agonist molecule.
3. The antagonist drug binds to the receptor and interrupts the sequence of events involved in an agonist activating the receptor.
4. The antagonist drug reduces the concentration of the active agonist molecule.
5. The bound antagonist response cancels the actions of the bound agonist response.

6. BIOCHEMISTRY

A. Acetyl-CoA
B. Aconitase
C. Citrate
D. Citrate synthase
E. Fumarate
F. Fumarate hydratase
G. Isocitrate
H. Isocitrate dehydrogenase
I. Malate
J. Malate dehydrogenase
K. Oxaloacetate
L. Oxoglutarate
M. Oxoglutarate dehydrogenase
N. Pyruvate
O. Pyruvate carboxylase
P. Succinate
Q. Succinate dehydrogenase
R. Succinyl-CoA

For each of the following descriptions, select the most appropriate molecule. Each option may be used once, more than once or not at all.

1. Acetyl-CoA is made from the conversion of this molecule.
2. Pyruvate is converted to oxaloacetate by this enzyme.
3. Acetyl-CoA is combined with this molecule.
4. This enzyme is responsible for forming isocitrate.
5. This intermediate in the Krebs cycle contains five carbons.

7. URINARY SYSTEM

A. Acute interstitial nephritis
B. Alport syndrome
C. Benign prostatic hyperplasia
D. Bladder carcinoma
E. Haemolytic–uraemic syndrome
F. Myoglobulinaemia
G. Renal artery stenosis
H. Schistosomiasis

For each of the following, select the appropriate condition. Each option may be used once, more than once or not at all.

1. This condition classically presents with painless haematuria.
2. This condition is a cause of squamous cell bladder cancer.
3. This condition is a cause of renal impairment and deafness.
4. This condition is a cause of brown urine and renal impairment.
5. This condition is a common cause of post-renal failure.

8. URINARY SYSTEM

A. Bence Jones proteins
B. Ethanol
C. Glucose
D. Ketones
E. Nitrates
F. Nitrites
G. Potassium
H. Red blood cells
I. Sodium
J. Urea
K. Urobilin

For each of the following, select the most appropriate biochemical finding. Each option may be used once, more than once or not at all.

1. Reabsorption at the proximal tubule is dependent on the movement of this solute.

2. This substance is found in the urine of a diabetic who has forgotten to take their insulin and presents with hyperventilation and sweet-smelling breath.
3. This substance might be found in the urine in someone with biliary obstruction.
4. This substance in the urine suggests myeloma.
5. This substance in the urine suggests infection.

9. URINARY SYSTEM

A. Aspirin overdose
B. Bulimia
C. Decreased anion gap
D. Depression
E. Diabetic ketoacidosis
F. Hyperthyroidism
G. Hyperventilation
H. Increased anion gap
I. Normal anion gap
J. Opiate overdose

The kidneys play a vital role in the regulation of acid–base balance. For each of the following, select the correct option from the list above. Each option may be used once, more than once or not at all.

1. This results in the respiratory compensation of metabolic acidosis.
2. This is a cause of metabolic alkalosis.
3. This is a cause of respiratory acidosis.
4. This is the effect of lactic acidosis on the anion gap.
5. This is the effect of renal tubular acidosis on the anion gap.

10. URINARY SYSTEM

A. Contrast nephropathy
B. Gentamicin therapy
C. Glomerulonephritis
D. Haematuria
E. Nephrotic syndrome
F. Pancreatitis
G. Polycystic kidney disease
H. Prostatic carcinoma

For each of the following scenarios, select the most likely cause of renal impairment. Each option may be used once, more than once or not at all.

1. This is the likely cause of intrinsic renal failure in a patient who recently underwent angiography for peripheral vascular disease.
2. This is pre-renal cause of uraemia.

3. This is a post-renal cause of uraemia.
4. This is an iatrogenic cause of intrinsic renal failure in a patient with septicaemia.
5. This is the likely cause of renal failure in a patient with systemic lupus erythematosus.

11. ORTHOPAEDICS AND RHEUMATOLOGY

A. Duchenne muscular dystrophy
B. Guillain–Barré syndrome
C. Huntington disease
D. Lambert–Eaton syndrome
E. Motor neuron disease
F. Multiple sclerosis
G. Myalgic encephalomyelitis
H. Myasthenia gravis
 I. Polymyalgia rheumatica
J. Rhabdomyolysis

For each of the following statements concerning the pathogenesis of muscle disease, select the correct condition. Each option may be used once, more than once or not at all.

1. This is a paraneoplastic condition, characterized by muscle weakness and absent tendon reflexes, commonly seen in patients with small cell lung cancer.
2. This is an autoimmune disease resulting in muscle 'fatigability'.
3. This is a demyelinating disease which can initially present with optic neuritis.
4. This is an acute infectious ascending polyneuropathy.
5. This is an autosomal dominant disorder resulting in progressive dementia and chorea.

12. ORTHOPAEDICS AND RHEUMATOLOGY

A. Acetylcholine receptor antibody
B. Anterior draw test
C. Anti-double-stranded DNA antibodies
D. Anti-glomerular antibodies
E. Creatinine
F. Cullen sign
G. Erythrocyte sedimentation rate
H. Glabellar tap sign
 I. Gowers sign
J. McMurray test
K. Oligoclonal bands
L. Phalen test
M. Xanthochromia

For each of the following, select the most appropriate marker, sign or test. Each option may be used once, more than once or not at all.

1. Which marker might be found in the cerebrospinal fluid of a patient with multiple sclerosis?
2. Which test is likely to be positive in a patient with carpal tunnel syndrome?
3. Which marker might be positive in a patient with myasthenia gravis?
4. Which marker is classically high in polymyalgia rheumatica?
5. Which sign might be evident in a child with Duchenne muscular dystrophy?

13. ORTHOPAEDICS AND RHEUMATOLOGY

A. Ankylosing spondylitis
B. Cushing syndrome
C. Dermatomyositis
D. Goodpasture syndrome
E. Polyarteritis nodosa
F. Polymyalgia rheumatica
G. Polymyositis
H. Rheumatoid arthritis
I. Systemic lupus erythematosus
J. Wegener granulomatosis

For each of the following statements, select the correct condition. Each option may be used once, more than once or not at all.

1. This is a cause of proximal myopathy, which can present with striae, bruising and acne.
2. This is a cause of enthesitis, a seronegative polyarthropathy, which usually presents in young men.
3. This is a cause of proximal muscle stiffness which presents in older people, classically with a high erythrocyte sedimentation rate.
4. This is a cause of proximal myopathy, which is a connective tissue disorder with a characteristic heliotrope rash and Gottron papules.
5. This is a cause of myalgia, an autoimmune multisystem disorder, classically with the presence of antinuclear and anti-double-stranded DNA antibodies.

14. ORTHOPAEDICS AND RHEUMATOLOGY

A. Biceps brachii
B. Common extensor tendon origin
C. Common flexor tendon origin
D. Deltoid
E. Lateral epicondylitis
F. Medial epicondylitis

G. Olecranon bursitis
H. Supraspinatus
 I. Trapezius
 J. Triceps brachii

For each of the following statements, select the correct condition or anatomical feature. Each option may be used once, more than once or not at all.

1. What is the medical term for 'tennis elbow'?
2. This is an alternative name for the medial epicondyle.
3. This is a muscle with three heads which facilitates elbow extension.
4. This is an inflammation of the common flexor origin.
5. This is a muscle of the rotator cuff.

15. ORTHOPAEDICS AND RHEUMATOLOGY
A. Adductor brevis
B. Adductor longus
C. Biceps femoris
D. Gastrocnemius
E. Gracilis
F. Peroneus longus
G. Piriformis
H. Psoas
 I. Rectus femoris
 J. Sartorius

For each of the following questions concerning muscles of the lower limb, select the correct option. Each option may be used once, more than once or not at all.

1. Which muscle is required in order to sit cross-legged?
2. Which muscle forms the medial border of the femoral triangle?
3. Which muscle is one of the hamstrings?
4. Which structure inserts into the Achilles tendon?
5. Which muscle is supplied by the femoral nerve to facilitate hip flexion and knee extension?

16. ORTHOPAEDICS AND RHEUMATOLOGY
A. Abductor pollicis brevis
B. Adductor pollicis brevis
C. Extensor carpi radialis longus
D. Flexor digitorum profundus
E. Flexor digitorum superficialis
F. Flexor pollicis brevis
G. Median nerve
H. Opponens pollicis

I. Radial nerve

J. Ulnar nerve

For each of the following concerning the anatomy of the hand, select the most appropriate option. Each option may be used once, more than once or not at all.

1. A 52-year-old woman with hypothyroidism presents with tingling and numbness of her hands. She has noticed weakness, particularly of her thumb. Which nerve is affected?
2. A 21-year-old man presents to his general practitioner with an injury to his finger sustained during a rugby match. He is unable to flex the distal interphalangeal (DIP) joint of his middle finger. Which tendon has he ruptured?
3. Which muscle of the thenar eminence is not supplied by the median nerve?
4. A 10-year-old boy presents to accident and emergency with his parents following a fall. An X-ray shows a left-sided humeral fracture. On examination he is unable to extend his left wrist. Which nerve has he damaged?
5. Which nerve supplies the medial one-and-a-half digits of the hand?

17. ORTHOPAEDICS AND RHEUMATOLOGY

A. Adductor longus
B. Anterior cruciate ligament
C. Biceps femoris
D. Deltoid ligament
E. Iliofemoral ligament
F. Ischiofemoral ligament
G. Lateral collateral ligament
H. Medial collateral ligament
I. Patellar tendon
J. Posterior cruciate ligament
K. Quadriceps tendon
L. Rectus femoris
M. Transverse ligament

For each of the following statements concerning the anatomy of the leg, select the most appropriate option. Each option may be used once, more than once or not at all.

1. This structure prevents anterior movement of the tibia in relation to the fibula.
2. The patella sits in this tendon as a sesamoid bone.
3. Stretching this elicits a reflex via nerve roots L3/L4.
4. Injury to this structure results in a 'sag' of the shin when the knee is flexed to 90 degree.
5. This contracts in response to the knee jerk reflex.

18. ORTHOPAEDICS AND RHEUMATOLOGY

A. Actin
B. Agonist
C. Antagonist
D. Cardiac muscle
E. Enthesitis
F. Epicondylitis
G. Ligament
H. Myosin
I. Skeletal muscle
J. Smooth muscle
K. Tendon

For each of the following questions, select the most appropriate option. Each option may be used once, more than once or not at all.

1. What is the name given to the thick filament of muscle fibres?
2. Which muscle type is composed of organized rows of fibres with a striated appearance?
3. What is the name of the structure connecting muscle to bone?
4. What is the action of triceps in elbow flexion?
5. What is the name given to inflammation at the site of tendon/ligament insertion?

19. ORTHOPAEDICS AND RHEUMATOLOGY

A. Achilles tendon
B. Anterior cruciate ligament
C. Biceps tendon
D. Brachioradialis
E. Gastrocnemius
F. Gluteus minimus
G. Lateral meniscus
H. Patellar tendon
I. Piriformis
J. Posterior cruciate ligament
K. Pre-patellar bursa
L. Pronator teres
M. Sacrotuberous ligaments

For each of the following, select the most appropriate option. Each option may be used once, more than once or not at all.

1. Which structure forms the lateral border of the cubital fossa?
2. Which structure prevents anterior dislocation of the knee?
3. Which structure inserts into the Achilles tendon?
4. Which of the above is involved in the L3/L4 tendon reflex?
5. Which of the above is involved in the L5/S1 tendon reflex?

20. ORTHOPAEDICS AND RHEUMATOLOGY

A. Barton fracture
B. Boxer's fracture
C. Colles fracture
D. March fracture
E. Pott's fracture
F. Salter–Harris fracture
G. Smith fracture
H. None of the above

For each of the following descriptions, select the most appropriate bone fracture. Each option may be used once, more than once or not at all.

1. This fracture involves the growth plate.
2. This fracture is sometimes called the dinner fork deformity.
3. This is a trimalleolar fracture of the ankle.
4. This is a fracture of the distal 5th metacarpal.
5. This is a fracture of the proximal ulna and dislocation of the ulna head.

Answers Paper 3

ANSWER QUESTION 1

1. C – Calcium channel blockers
Either a calcium channel blocker (amlodipine most commonly) or a thiazide diuretic can be used as first-line management. There is a variation in the selection between black and non-black patients under the age of 55 due to the response to treatment with ACE inhibitors. It has been observed that black people tend to respond less well to treatment with ACE inhibitors than non-black patients. This is likely related to the low renin state in this patient group. Non-black patients under the age of 55 should be treated with an ACE inhibitor as first-line therapy unless there is a good contraindication.

2. A – Angiotensin-converting enzyme inhibitors
ACE inhibitors are extremely good in the treatment of hypertension in non-black patients. They are the first line management for non-black patients under the age of 55. If optimal blood pressure is not achieved with an ACE inhibitor titrated to a maximal dose, a second therapy should be added. Second-line treatments in this group of patients include the addition of either a calcium channel blocker or a thiazide diuretic.

3. C – Calcium channel blockers
In this instance, a calcium channel blocker would be most appropriate. A relatively common drug to start with would be amlodipine 5 mg daily. Thiazide diuretics have been shown to impair uric acid excretion and can occasionally result in gout. Patients with a past medical history of gout should therefore not be started on a thiazide diuretic, as this may precipitate an acute episode.

4. G – Minoxidil
Minoxidil is not commonly used for hypertension; however, it is extremely useful for patients with severe hypertension requiring inpatient control. This drug is a potent antihypertensive which exerts its effects through vasodilation. Minoxidil is given as a continuous intravenous infusion, and patients should be weaned off slowly. Abruptly stopping minoxidil can result in rebound hypertension.

5. B – Beta-blockers
Beta-blockers are associated quite commonly with vivid dreams, nightmares and hallucinations. Alongside these unpleasant side-effects, patients

may also suffer with low mood, poor exercise tolerance and erectile problems. It is important to warn patients of these side-effects before starting them on these drugs.

There are current guidelines available from the National Institute for Health and Clinical Excellence (NICE) and the British Hypertension Society providing important information regarding the evidence-based treatment of hypertension.

ANSWER QUESTION 2

1. H – Verapamil

Verapamil is absolutely contraindicated in patients with Wolff–Parkinson–White syndrome. Patients may present with a fast, broad complex tachycardia. On initial glance, this may look like ventricular tachycardia (VT), and patients may be incorrectly given a dose of verapamil. A patient with an accessory pathway and atrial fibrillation (AF) may conduct through the accessory pathway. This is known as AF with aberrant conduction. On closer inspection, it becomes apparent that the rate is not regular, which helps to differentiate it from VT. By giving a patient verapamil, all conduction through the normal conduction system is blocked, resulting in uninhibited transmission of AF through the accessory pathway. Patients may subsequently degenerate into ventricular fibrillation.

2. B – Amiodarone

Amiodarone is a classic exam question subject. It has a host of side-effects, including slate-grey skin, photosensitive rashes, corneal micro-deposits and pulmonary fibrosis. Abnormalities of thyroid function may also occur.

3. C – Bisoprolol

Despite digoxin being the drug that people often use, NICE guidelines state that the first-line management for rate control of AF is beta-blockers, followed by calcium channel blockers. Third-line management is digoxin. The major problem with digoxin is rate control during exercise. Patients can be rate-controlled at rest, but as soon as they brush their teeth or walk up the stairs, their rate goes back up to 120 bpm. Digoxin does have its place as a first-line management, but this is often in older patients with extremely limited exercise tolerances.

4. A – Adenosine

Adenosine can be used to create a transient atrioventricular (AV) block. As a result it is particularly useful in patients with supraventricular tachycardias (SVTs). The temporary AV block can terminate SVTs; however, carotid sinus massage and vagal manoeuvres should be tried prior to the administration of adenosine. Fast rhythms confined to the atria or ventricles that do not involve the AV node as part of the re-entry circuit cannot be terminated with adenosine; however, the transient AV block may reveal the underlying rhythm.

5. B – Amiodarone

Disorders of thyroid function occur in approximately 15%–20% of patients treated with amiodarone. The most common thyroid disorder is thyrotoxicosis, but amiodarone-induced hypothyroidism is also encountered. These disturbances in thyroid function are due to amiodarone being an iodine-rich drug.

ANSWER QUESTION 3

1. D – Enalapril

Enalapril is an angiotensin converting enzyme (ACE) inhibitor. ACE is produced in the lungs and converts angiotensin I to angiotensin II, which raises blood pressure by vasoconstriction and stimulating aldosterone release. Aldosterone is secreted from the adrenal cortex to facilitate water and sodium retention. Its pressor effects, along with fluid retention, result in an increase in blood pressure. By blocking the renin–angiotensin–aldosterone (RAA) pathway, the ACE inhibitors are effective in the management of hypertension. A dry cough is a common side-effect. Patients who cannot tolerate the side-effects can be given an angiotensin II receptor blocker (e.g. losartan) as an alternative.

2. I – Spironolactone

Spironolactone is an aldosterone antagonist used in the management of hypertension. Aldosterone is released from the adrenal cortex in response to activation of the RAA pathway. It increases blood pressure by promoting salt and water retention and by vasoconstriction, thus increasing vascular resistance. Gynaecomastia, the development of extensive breast tissue in men, commonly occurs with spironolactone.

3. F – Furosemide

Furosemide is a loop diuretic commonly used in the management of hypertension, congestive cardiac failure and oedema. The loop diuretics act on the $Na^+/K^+/2Cl^-$ cotransporter to inhibit salt reabsorption, which results in diuresis. Potassium is also lost and so loop diuretics predispose to hypokalaemia. When given parenterally at a high dose, furosemide can prove ototoxic leading to deafness.

4. B – Bendroflumethiazide

Bendroflumethiazide belongs to the group of thiazide diuretics, creating diuresis by inhibiting sodium reabsorption at the proximal convoluted tubule. Side-effects include hypokalaemia, dehydration (particularly in the elderly), hyperuricaemia and gout. Other examples of thiazides include indapamide and metolazone.

5. H – Mannitol

Mannitol is an osmotic diuretic used in the treatment of cerebral oedema and for raised intraocular pressure (i.e. glaucoma). Mannitol is filtered by the glomeruli but is not reabsorbed and so creates an osmotic drive which reduces sodium and water reabsorption, and thus reduces extracellular volume. Its side-effects include thrombophlebitis, oedema and angina-like chest pains, although these are all relatively rare.

ANSWER QUESTION 4

1. F – They inhibit translocation
2. B – They affect DNA gyrase
3. A – They affect anticodon recognition, which leads to the misreading of the DNA
4. B – They affect DNA gyrase
5. G – They inhibit transpeptidation

Macrolides inhibit translocation by binding reversibly to the subunit 50S of the bacterial ribosome. Tetracyclines compete with tRNA for the A site. Sulphonamides affect folate synthesis. Fluoroquinolones inhibit topoisomerase II, which is a DNA gyrase. Aminoglycosides cause anticodon recognition, which leads to the misreading of the DNA. Beta-lactams interfere with the bacterial cell wall peptidoglycan synthesis. Chloramphenicol inhibits transpeptidation. Puromycin causes premature termination of the peptide chain.

ANSWER QUESTION 5

1. A – Chemical antagonism

Chemical antagonism describes a situation where the antagonist drug reacts with the agonist molecule in such a way that the agonist molecule is no longer able to either occupy and/or activate its target receptor to elicit a response.

2. B – Competitive antagonism

In competitive antagonism, both the antagonist drug and the agonist molecule compete for the same target binding site. When the antagonist drug binds, the target is not activated – hence antagonism. A given concentration of an antagonist drug will reduce the number of target sites occupied by the agonist molecule. In competitive antagonism, the apparent affinity of the agonist is reduced.

3. E – Non-competitive antagonism

When an agonist occupies and activates its target protein, there is a cascade of events that lead to the production of a functional response. In non-competitive antagonism, the drug antagonist binds elsewhere to the target protein, and though it does not prevent the agonist molecule from binding, in some way it interrupts the cascade of events that lead to the response. Thus, no response is elicited and the active agonist is antagonized.

4. F – Pharmacokinetic antagonism

Pharmacokinetic antagonism is when the antagonist drug decreases the concentration of the active agonist, thus preventing agonist occupancy of target receptors and their consequent response. Thus, it antagonizes active molecules. The antagonist drug can reduce active agonist concentrations by affecting its metabolism or excretion.

5. G – Physiological antagonism

Physiological antagonism describes a situation where the antagonist drug occupies and activates a receptor to elicit a response that opposes and cancels out the response elicited by an agonist molecule.

ANSWER QUESTION 6

1. N – Pyruvate

Acetyl-CoA is made from the conversion of pyruvate. Pyruvate is the endpoint of the process called glycolysis. Acetyl-CoA can also be obtained by other processes such as breakdown of fatty acid as well as the carbon skeletons of some amino acids.

2. O – Pyruvate carboxylase

Pyruvate carboxylase is an enzyme which is responsible for converting pyruvate into oxaloacetate, a four-carbon compound that is an important molecule in the Krebs cycle.

3. K – Oxaloacetate

Oxaloacetate is a four-carbon compound. It is combined with acetyl-CoA, a two-carbon compound, by the enzyme citrate synthase to form a six-carbon compound citrate.

4. B – Aconitase

Citrate is a six-carbon compound in the citric acid cycle. It is acted on by the enzyme aconitase. Aconitase removes a water molecule from citrate to form *cis*-aconitase; it then adds a water molecule to *cis*-aconitase to form isocitrate.

5. L – Oxoglutarate

Oxoglutarate is a five-carbon compound found in the Krebs cycle. It is formed from a six-carbon molecule isocitrate, which is converted to oxoglutarate via the enzyme isocitrate dehydrogenase. During the conversion of isocitrate to oxoglutarate, CO_2 and NADH are formed and leave the Krebs cycle. This results in oxoglutarate, a five-carbon compound which has been made from the enzymatic conversion of a six-carbon compound.

ANSWER QUESTION 7

1. D – Bladder carcinoma

Over 95% of cases of bladder cancer originate in the transitional cell. It classically presents with painless haematuria. Other causes of haematuria include calculi, renal cell carcinoma and polycystic kidney disease, but they normally have an element of pain. Risk factors for developing bladder cancer include occupational exposure to dyes, schistosomiasis infection and smoking.

2. H – Schistosomiasis

Schistosomiasis infection can cause bladder cancer, but of the squamous type. Although rare in the UK, its incidence is higher in areas where schistosomiasis is prevalent, such as most of Africa and parts of South America. This parasitic infection is also known as bilharzia. It presents with cough, diarrhoea, abdominal pain, hepatosplenomegaly and genital lesions, which increase the risk of contracting HIV.

3. B – Alport syndrome

Alport syndrome is an inherited disorder with a variable inheritance pattern and is characterized by sensorineural deafness, visual disturbance and progressive renal failure. The defect is in type IV collagen and results in damage to the glomerular basement membrane. End-stage renal failure normally develops before the age of 30 and transplantation is required.

4. F – Myoglobulinaemia

Myoglobulinaemia occurs as a product of muscle breakdown. Rhabdomyolysis causes myoglobin release. Myoglobin can accumulate in the tubules and reduces renal function. The myoglobin that is excreted turns the urine dark. Causes of rhabdomyolysis include falls, disuse, crush injuries, MDMA (3,4-methylenedioxymethamphetamine, commonly known as ecstasy), poisoning and malignant hyperthermia.

5. C – Benign prostatic hyperplasia

Post-renal failure occurs with obstruction of the urinary tract somewhere between the renal calyces to the external urethral sphincter. Benign prostatic hyperplasia is a common cause in older men. They may present with symptoms of hesitancy, poor stream and terminal dribbling. Alpha antagonists (e.g. doxazosin) can help to relax the smooth muscle and reduce symptoms, while finasteride inhibits testosterone metabolism, which reduces prostatic size.

ANSWER QUESTION 8

1. I – Sodium

The active transport of sodium at the proximal tubule facilitates the reabsorption of many other solutes. These include glucose, electrolytes and amino acids. There are many sodium transporters including the Na+–glucose cotransporter, the Na+–Cl- transporter and the Na+–H+ exchanger. The proximal tubule is highly permeable to water and reabsorption is isotonic in this region of the nephron.

2. D – Ketones

Diabetic ketoacidosis often occurs along with intercurrent illness. The patient may not be eating and thus have stopped taking insulin. Alternatively, it may be the first presentation of diabetes mellitus in a child. Symptoms include extreme thirst, polyuria, nausea and vomiting. The acidosis induces hyperventilation (Kussmaul breathing), as the body tries to 'blow off' acid in the form of carbon dioxide. Drowsiness can lead to reduced consciousness and coma. Treatment is with insulin and fluid replacement. Care must be taken not to replace circulating volume too rapidly, as cerebral oedema can result.

3. K – Urobilin

Biliary obstruction can be the result of a common bile duct gallstone or a tumour at the head of the pancreas. Characteristically there is dark urine and pale stools. Unconjugated bilirubin is the product of erythrocyte breakdown. It is transferred to the liver for conjugation. In obstruction, less conjugated bilirubin is released into the gut via the ampulla of Vater. Consequently, there is less urobilinogen formation in the gut. Under normal circumstances, some of the urobilinogen is reabsorbed and excreted by the kidney as urobilin. High levels of conjugated bilirubin in the blood are renally excreted and give urine its dark colour. Limited amounts of urobilinogen in the gut mean that less stercobilin is present in faeces, resulting in pale stools.

4. A – Bence Jones proteins

Myeloma results from the uncontrolled proliferation of plasma cells. Plasma cells produce the monoclonal immunoglobulin paraprotein. Symptoms include bone pain, malaise and weight loss. Bone destruction causes osteolytic appearances on X-ray, hypercalcaemia and recurrent fractures. Light chains accumulate and precipitate renal failure. These light chains are often present in urine as Bence Jones proteins. Other investigation results include a high erythrocyte sedimentation rate (ESR), high levels of plasma cells in the bone marrow and an M-band on protein electrophoresis.

5. F – Nitrites

Urinary tract infection is very common, particularly in pregnancy, diabetes and the elderly. Urine dipsticks can be used to detect infection. Most bacterial species (*Escherichia coli* being the most common) causing urinary infection convert urinary nitrates to nitrites and these are detected on the dipstick test. Leucocyte esterase, blood and protein are also detected. The sample must always be sent off for microscopy and culture, and to check antibiotic sensitivities.

ANSWER QUESTION 9

1. G – Hyperventilation

An acidosis can be compensated by respiratory and renal means. A metabolic acidosis can be compensated by increasing the rate of breathing. Hyperventilating allows carbon dioxide to be blown off, increasing the $HCO_3^- : CO_2$ ratio which, according to the Henderson–Hasselbalch equation, increases the pH:

$$pH = pK_a + \log\left(\frac{HCO_3^-}{CO_2}\right)$$

pK_a = the acid dissociation constant

2. B – Bulimia

Metabolic alkalosis results in an increase in pH because of increased plasma bicarbonate or chloride, or decreased hydrogen or potassium ions. Common causes of metabolic alkalosis in hospital include vomiting, the use of diuretics (e.g. furosemide) and nasogastric suction. Other rarer causes include cystic fibrosis, Conn's syndrome (primary hyperaldosteronism) and villous adenoma. Vomiting and bulimia result in gastric HCl loss and a subsequent metabolic alkalosis.

3. J – Opiate overdose

Respiratory acidosis results in a decrease in pH because of carbon dioxide retention. This may be secondary to hypoventilation or poor gaseous exchange at the alveoli. Opiate overdose results in respiratory depression. This may be a heroin overdose in an intravenous drug abuser or iatrogenic, owing to excess morphine or codeine given in the hospital setting. In addition to respiratory depression, opiate overdose results in bilateral pupillary constriction, drowsiness and ultimately coma. Naloxone is given to reverse the effects of opiate toxicity.

4. H – Increased anion gap

The anion gap is extremely useful in assessing the cause of a metabolic acidosis and can be calculated using the formula:

$$\text{Anion gap} = \left(\left[Na^+\right]+\left[K^+\right]\right)-\left(\left[HCO_3^-\right]+\left[Cl^-\right]\right)$$

Because there are more positive ions (anions) than negative ions (cations), the normal range of the anion gap is 10–18 mmol/L. If the anion gap is increased, it can be deduced that the metabolic acidosis is caused by the presence of unmeasured anions. Causes of a metabolic acidosis with a high anion gap include lactic acidosis, diabetic ketoacidosis and aspirin overdose.

5. I – Normal anion gap

Causes of metabolic acidosis with a normal anion gap include renal tubular acidosis and diarrhoea. Renal tubular acidosis (RTA) results in a decrease in plasma pH and may be secondary to structural, immunological or drug-induced tubular damage. It is divided into four different types: type 1 (distal RTA) results from a failure in H⁺ secretion at the distal tubule; type 2 (proximal RTA) results in failure of HCO_3^- reabsorption at the proximal tubule; type 3 (inherited RTA) is very rare and results in a combination of types 1 and 2; finally, type 4, the most common type of RTA, is characterized by low renin and aldosterone and results in hyperkalaemic acidosis.

ANSWER QUESTION 10

1. A – Contrast nephropathy
Contrast nephropathy can occur following contrast imaging and results in an increase in serum creatinine by 25%. Conditions predisposing to contrast nephropathy include reduced circulating volume, diabetes mellitus and pre-existing renal disease.

2. F – Pancreatitis
Pancreatitis can result in pre-renal failure owing to third space fluid loss. This results in reduced renal perfusion. Acute pancreatitis should be managed with intravenous rehydration, analgesia and occasionally antibiotics. Other causes of pre-renal failure include anything that can reduce circulating volume (e.g. haemorrhage or dehydration) or reduce cardiac output and blood pressure (e.g. left ventricular failure).

3. H – Prostatic carcinoma
Prostatic carcinoma can result in obstruction of the urethra. Obstructive uropathy results in post-renal failure, which can be caused by renal calculi, pelvic tumours or blood clots. Prostatic carcinoma may be felt on rectal examination as a hard, rough, irregularly shaped prostate, with loss of the central sulcus. A transrectal ultrasound and biopsy can confirm diagnosis. Prostate-specific antigen can be used to monitor response to treatment.

4. B – Gentamicin therapy
Aminoglycosides, such as gentamicin, are excreted primarily by the kidneys, which causes levels to accumulate in renal impairment. For this reason, the once-daily high-dose regimen should be avoided in patients with renal impairment. Serum gentamicin levels must be monitored, and renal, auditory and vestibular function regularly assessed. The important side-effects of the aminoglycosides include ototoxicity and nephrotoxicity.

5. C – Glomerulonephritis
Systemic lupus erythematosus (SLE) is a multisystem disease in which 40% of patients have some renal involvement. This may present as asymptomatic proteinuria, nephritic syndrome or rapid renal failure. The different types of lupus nephritis range from minimal mesangial

glomerulonephritis to advanced sclerosing nephritis. Steroids and immu-nosuppressive agents are used, but prognosis depends on the stage of renal disease and the level of pre-existing histological damage.

ANSWER QUESTION 11

1. D – Lambert–Eaton syndrome

Lambert–Eaton syndrome is a paraneoplastic condition which commonly (in 50% of cases) occurs in small-cell carcinoma of the lungs. It is a myas-thenia-like condition with proximal muscle weakness, causing defective acetylcholine release at the neuromuscular junction. There is sometimes ocular and bulbar involvement, and tendon reflexes are typically absent. The pathogenesis is thought to involve antibodies against voltage-gated calcium channels, which are found in 90% of cases.

2. H – Myasthenia gravis

Myasthenia gravis is an autoimmune disease caused by auto-antibodies against the acetylcholine receptors on the postsynaptic membrane at the neuromuscular junction. This results in gradual decline in muscle func-tion and the characteristic symptom of 'fatigability'. Extraocular and bul-bar muscles are commonly affected. Acetylcholinesterase inhibitors (e.g. neostigmine) are used to prevent the breakdown of acetylcholine and thus improve muscle function. Myasthenia gravis commonly occurs alongside other autoimmune conditions, which include pernicious anaemia, Graves disease and vitiligo.

3. F – Multiple sclerosis

Multiple sclerosis is a demyelinating disorder of unknown cause which leads to reduced nervous transmission. Demyelination occurs at different locations and at different times. Although disease progression varies, the disorder commonly occurs in a relapsing-and-remitting manner. The optic nerve is commonly affected, particularly early on in the disease, and patients typically present with transient unilateral visual loss, which may be associated with pain. Sensory impairment is common with paraesthe-siae and numbness.

4. B – Guillain–Barré syndrome

Guillain–Barré syndrome is an ascending inflammatory polyneuropathy, which commonly presents 2–3 weeks following a respiratory or gastro-intestinal infection. The cause is unknown, but there is thought to be an element of demyelination. Paraesthesiae and ascending limb weakness are classical symptoms, although bulbar and respiratory involvement can occur.

5. C – Huntington disease

Huntington disease is a neurodegenerative disorder resulting from repeat CAG sequences in the Huntington gene. It is inherited in an autosomal dominant manner and is characterized by progressive dementia and chorea. Degeneration is particularly marked in the caudate nucleus of the basal ganglia. Age of onset is usually 35–40 and death commonly occurs within 15 years.

ANSWER QUESTION 12

1. K – Oligoclonal bands

Oligoclonal bands are immunoglobulins deposited in the CSF or serum which are seen on protein electrophoresis. Multiple sclerosis is a demyelinating disease that results in reduced neuronal transmission velocity. It is more common in women and typically presents with an episode of optic neuritis, which is characterized by transient loss of vision. The disease tends to relapse and remit, although some cases are progressive whereby there is a gradual decline in function.

2. L – Phalen test

Phalen test can be used in the diagnosis of carpal tunnel syndrome. By asking the patient to flex the wrist by pressing the dorsum of the hands together, the median nerve is compressed in the carpal tunnel. The test is positive when the symptoms of carpal tunnel syndrome are reproduced. Conditions that predispose to carpal tunnel syndrome include rheumatoid arthritis, pregnancy and hypothyroidism.

3. A – Acetylcholine receptor antibody

Myasthenia gravis is a disease of reduced neuromuscular transmission which results in 'fatigability'. It is an autoimmune condition with auto-antibodies against the acetylcholine receptor. The disease can be managed with acetylcholinesterase inhibitors, and thymectomy is commonly performed because of the close correlation between thymic pathology and myasthenia gravis.

4. G – Erythrocyte sedimentation rate

Polymyalgia rheumatica is a geriatric condition resulting in stiffness of the proximal muscles. There is usually pain and limitation of movement. It is thought to be pathologically linked to giant cell (temporal) arteritis in which inflammation of the temporal artery can result in blindness. Both conditions respond to steroid therapy. Care must be taken to prevent adrenal suppression and Addisonian crisis on withdrawal of the medication.

5. I – Gowers sign

Duchenne muscular dystrophy is caused by mutations to the dystrophin gene on the X chromosome and affects approximately 1 in 3500 male births. It typically presents with delayed motor milestones and delayed speech. Gowers sign is when a child with Duchenne muscular dystrophy attempts to stand from a sitting position. They will use their hands to 'walk up' their legs in order to stand. The condition has a poor prognosis with death commonly occurring from cardio-respiratory failure in the 20s.

ANSWER QUESTION 13

1. B – Cushing syndrome
Cushing syndrome results from excess cortisol, which can be iatrogenic via exogenous steroids, or secondary to an adrenocorticotropic hormone (ACTH)-secreting tumour (Cushing disease). It is characterized by proximal myopathy, centripetal fat distribution and, classically, if not rather unkindly, patients are described as having a 'buffalo hump' and 'moon face'. Other signs of excess cortisol include acne, striae and bruising. Patients are frequently hypertensive.

2. A – Ankylosing spondylitis
Ankylosing spondylitis presents in young men, typically between 20 and 40 years old. It is a seronegative (i.e. rheumatoid factor negative) arthropathy in which patients complain of stiffness and pain in the back which improves with exercise. Patients are classically said to have a 'question mark posture', with hyperextension of the neck to compensate for flexion of the upper spine. Enthesitis describes the inflammation of the site at which tendons attach to bone, which is a common finding in ankylosing spondylitis.

3. F – Polymyalgia rheumatica
Polymyalgia rheumatica is a disease of older people (typically over 60 years), which results in stiffness and pain of the girdle muscles. The ESR is usually high, and the condition responds well to steroid treatment. Care must be taken to taper the steroid dose and not abruptly stop the drug, to prevent adrenal suppression and Addisonian crisis.

4. C – Dermatomyositis
Dermatomyositis is a connective tissue disorder resulting in proximal myopathy, as in polymyositis, but with additional skin involvement. It presents with a characteristic rash on the knuckles (Gottron papules) and a heliotrope rash of the eyelids. Calcification of muscles can occur, as can interstitial pulmonary fibrosis.

5. I – Systemic lupus erythematosus
Systemic lupus erythematosus (SLE) is a multisystem disorder that can result in disease of the musculoskeletal system (e.g. small joint arthropathy), kidneys (e.g. lupus glomerulonephritis), heart (e.g. endocarditis), lungs (e.g. interstitial fibrosis), brain (e.g. cerebrovascular disease) and skin (e.g. malar/butterfly rash). This autoimmune connective tissue disorder is more common in women and tends to present between 20 and 40 years of age. Both ANA (antinuclear) and anti-dsDNA (anti-double strand DNA) antibodies are raised in some cases. The condition tends to

relapse and remit, and so management involves addressing the current symptoms. Corticosteroids and immunosuppressants are used in managing active SLE.

ANSWER QUESTION 14

1. E – Lateral epicondylitis
Lateral epicondylitis is also known as 'tennis elbow' (remember the two 't's). It is characterized by tenderness on palpation of the lateral epicondyle and on wrist extension. Classically, it results from activities using wrist extension (e.g. playing tennis). Management consists of non-steroidal anti-inflammatory drugs, cold compress, rest and physiotherapy.

2. C – Common flexor tendon origin
The medial epicondyle is the site of attachment of the common tendon of the forearm flexors, which include the pronator teres, flexor carpi radialis, palmaris longus and flexor digitorum superficialis. It is therefore known as the common flexor tendon origin. Inflammation over this site, medial epicondylitis, is known as 'golfer's elbow', resulting in pain on wrist flexion and tenderness on palpation of the medial epicondyle.

3. J – Triceps brachii
The triceps brachii is a three-headed muscle responsible for shoulder extension, adduction and the elbow extension. It is innervated by the radial nerve, which supplies the forearm extensors. The triceps tendon reflex is innervated by C7/8 and may be exaggerated in upper motor neuron lesions and reduced or dampened in lower motor neuron disease.

4. F – Medial epicondylitis
The common flexor origin is the medial epicondyle and the site of attachment of the forearm flexors. Inflammation at this bony prominence results in tenderness to palpation and pain on wrist flexion (classically, after playing golf).

5. H – Supraspinatus
The rotator cuff muscles comprise the supraspinatus, infraspinatus, teres minor and subscapularis ('sits'). They stabilize the glenohumeral joint and facilitate rotation and abduction. The teres minor and infraspinatus allow lateral rotation of the joint, while the subscapularis initiates medial rotation. Finally, the supraspinatus facilitates abduction.

ANSWER QUESTION 15

1. J – Sartorius
The sartorius, meaning 'tailor-like', is required in order to sit cross-legged. It is supplied by the femoral nerve and facilitates hip and knee flexion in addition to lateral rotation at the hip. Along with the sartorius,

the femoral nerve also supplies the four quadriceps muscles and pectineus, which extend the knee and flex the hip, respectively.

2. B – Adductor longus

The femoral triangle contains the femoral nerve, artery and vein and is bordered by the inguinal ligament (superiorly), the adductor longus (medially) and the sartorius (laterally). As its name suggests, the adductor longus is responsible for adduction at the hip, as well as medial rotation. Along with the other adductors, it is supplied by the obturator nerve.

3. C – Biceps femoris

The hamstring muscles are the biceps femoris, semitendinosus and semimembranosus. They are the muscles of the posterior compartment of the lower limb and bring about hip extension and knee flexion. They are supplied by the sciatic nerve, which may be damaged in posterior hip dislocation or intramuscular injection in the buttocks.

4. D – Gastrocnemius

The gastrocnemius is the largest of the calf muscles and inserts into the Achilles tendon, along with the soleus and plantaris. It is supplied by the tibial nerve (a branch of the sciatic nerve) and is responsible for knee flexion and plantar flexion.

5. I – Rectus femoris

The rectus femoris, vastus medialis, vastus intermedius and vastus lateralis make up the quadriceps muscles. They are supplied by the femoral nerve and facilitate knee extension and hip flexion. The rectus femoris arises from two tendons: one attaches to the anterior superior iliac spine and the other to the acetabulum. The quadriceps muscles are the direct antagonists to the hamstring muscles, which consist of the biceps femoris, semitendinosus and semimembranosus.

ANSWER QUESTION 16

1. G – Median nerve

Carpal tunnel syndrome results from compression of the median nerve as it traverses through the carpal tunnel between the carpal bones and the flexor retinaculum. It is characterized by weakness, pain and paraesthesia of the hands. Sensory loss of the lateral three-and-a-half digits can also occur. Conditions that predispose to carpal tunnel syndrome include diabetes, hypothyroidism, rheumatoid arthritis and pregnancy. Surgery can be performed to release the entrapment.

2. D – Flexor digitorum profundus

The flexor digitorum profundus (FDP) attaches to the base of the distal phalanx and is therefore responsible for flexion at the distal interphalangeal (DIP) joint. The flexor digitorum superficialis (FDS) terminates at the middle phalanx and so plays a part in flexion of the proximal interphalangeal (PIP) joint. Rupture of the FDP is a relatively common sports injury caused by pulling on an opponent's shirt while they are running away. Forced extension of the joint during active flexion results in rupture of the tendon.

3. B – Adductor pollicis brevis
The majority of the small muscles of the hand are supplied by the ulnar nerve. The four muscles supplied by the median nerve can be remembered by the acronym LOAF:

*L*ateral two lumbricals
*O*pponens pollicis
*A*bductor pollicis brevis
*F*lexor pollicis brevis

The radial nerve supplies the wrist extensors (extensor carpi radialis, extensor carpi ulnaris).

4. I – Radial nerve
The radial nerve is vulnerable to trauma as it winds around the shaft of the humerus. Fractures here can damage the nerve, resulting in the classical presentation of wrist drop, because the radial nerve supplies the extensors. Another cause of radial nerve palsy is 'Saturday night palsy', whereby the nerve gets compressed by falling asleep with the arm draped over the back of the sofa.

5. J – Ulnar nerve
The ulnar nerve supplies sensation to the medial one-and-a-half digits, while the lateral three-and-a-half digits are supplied by the median nerve. (Remember the anatomy is described as if the patient was standing in the anatomical position, i.e. the thenar eminence is most lateral and the hypothenar most medial.) The radial nerve has only a limited sensory component and supplies the first web space on the dorsum of the hand.

ANSWER QUESTION 17

1. B – Anterior cruciate ligament
The anterior cruciate ligament (ACL) is one of the four ligaments that stabilize the femorotibial joint. From the femur it attaches to the intercondylar eminence of the tibia and prevents anterior movement of the tibia in relation to the femur. Damage can result from twisting injuries to the knee, causing pain, occasional haemarthrosis and joint instability. The anterior draw test is classically positive; ligament laxity allows the tibia to be pulled forward with respect to the fibula. Magnetic resonance imaging (MRI) is the investigation of choice.

2. K – Quadriceps tendon
The patella sits in the quadriceps tendon as a sesamoid bone, anterior to the knee joint. It articulates with the femoral condyles. It is thought to act

as a pulley to improve movement at the joint. The knee is a synovial hinge joint stabilized by four ligaments: anterior and posterior cruciates, and lateral and medial collateral ligaments. The medial and lateral menisci improve articulation.

3. I – Patellar tendon

The patellar tendon reflex is innervated by the nerve roots L3/L4. Upon stretching of the tendon, muscle spindles are activated and send afferent signals via the nerve fibres. Efferents, via the α-motor neuron, result in contraction of rectus femoris and extension of the knee. Other important reflexes to know are the ankle jerk reflex (L5/S1), brachial reflex (C5/C6) and triceps reflex (C6/C7).

4. J – Posterior cruciate ligament

The posterior cruciate ligament (PCL) prevents posterior movement of the tibia with respect to the femur. Injury results in a positive posterior drawer test, in which the tibia 'sags' backwards when the knee is flexed to 90 degree. The PCL is thicker and stronger than the ACL, and so is less prone to injury than the ACL.

5. L – Rectus femoris

The knee jerk reflex results in contraction of rectus femoris via L3/L4 nerve roots. The rectus femoris is a muscle of the quadriceps responsible for knee extension and hip flexion. The quadriceps is supplied by the femoral nerve and comprises the vastus medialis, vastus intermedius and vastus lateralis. The hamstrings elicit the opposite movement and are supplied by the sciatic nerve.

ANSWER QUESTION 18

1. H – Myosin

Striated or skeletal muscle is composed of myofibrils, which are divided into sarcomeres. Muscle contraction is brought about by the action of two filaments, myosin and actin. Myosin filaments are thicker than actin filaments and the two are arranged so that they interdigitate with one another. The degree of overlap determines the force of contraction. Increasing initial muscle stretch up to an optimal length increases the force of contraction. If the fibre is stretched beyond this length, the actin and myosin filaments are pulled too far apart and cross-bridge formation cannot occur.

2. I – Skeletal muscle

Skeletal muscle is organized in a striated fashion, with dark and light bands. The dark bands result from overlap of the myosin and actin filaments, while the lighter bands contain only actin. Contraction takes place via ATP-dependent cross-bridge formation in the following stages:

- ATP binds to the myosin head group.
- Actin dissociates from myosin.

- ATP → ADP + phosphate.
- The myosin head group pivots so that it is at a 90° angle to the actin filaments.
- The myosin head group binds to actin.
- The release of Pi causes the 'power stroke', by which the myosin head pivots through 45°, moving the actin with respect to the myosin.
- ADP is released to complete and restart the cycle.

3. K – Tendon

Ligaments classically describe the connective tissue structure that joins bone to bone, while tendons attach bone to muscle. Simple examples include the inguinal ligament, which joins the anterior superior iliac spine (ASIS) and the pubic tubercle, and the quadriceps tendon, which attaches the hip flexors (quadriceps femoris) to the patella.

4. C – Antagonist

Elbow flexion is brought about by contraction of the biceps brachii, brachioradialis, brachialis and coracobrachialis. They are therefore the elbow flexion agonists. The antagonist works to oppose this movement, and thus contraction results in elbow extension. The antagonist to elbow flexion is therefore the triceps muscle, which is supplied by the radial nerve.

5. E – Enthesitis

Enthesitis is inflammation of the site of attachment of tendon or ligaments. A common condition predisposing to enthesitis is ankylosing spondylitis. Ankylosing spondylitis is a seronegative arthropathy that is most common in young men. Patients complain of pain and stiffness in the back which is typically worse in the morning and improved with exercise (cf. osteoarthritis back pain, which is worse at night).

ANSWER QUESTION 19

1. D – Brachioradialis

The cubital fossa is a region on the anterior surface of the elbow joint. Its floor is formed by the supinators and the roof by fascia and skin. It is a triangular region bordered by brachioradialis laterally, pronator teres medially with its base formed by a line between the lateral and medial epicondyles of the humerus. Within the cubital fossa, the brachial artery can be palpated medial to the prominent biceps tendon. The median nerve also passes through the fossa as it runs to the hand to supply lateral sensation and muscles of the thenar eminence.

2. B – Anterior cruciate ligament

The anterior cruciate ligament acts to prevent anterior movement of the tibia with respect to the femur. Laxity of the ligament can be demonstrated with the anterior drawer test, in which the tibia can be pulled forwards on the femur. Other structures acting to protect and stabilize the knee joint include the posterior cruciate, medial and lateral collaterals, the menisci and bursae.

3. E – Gastrocnemius
The gastrocnemius is the most prominent muscle of the calf, responsible for knee flexion. It inserts into the Achilles tendon, which also allows the gastrocnemius to facilitate plantar flexion, along with flexor digitorum longus, tibialis posterior, soleus and flexor hallucis longus. The gastrocnemius is supplied by the tibial nerve.

4. H – Patellar tendon
The patellar or knee jerk reflex is brought about via nerve roots L3/L4. Stretching of the patellar tendon results in activation of a spinal reflex pathway. This causes contraction of the rectus femoris and extension of the knee. Reflex testing is an important part of a neuromuscular examination. Increased or exaggerated reflexes suggest an upper motor neuron pathology, although it may be caused by hyperthyroidism or even excess caffeine.

5. A – Achilles tendon
The ankle jerk reflex is a reflex pathway of roots L5/S1. Stretching the Achilles tendon results in the reflex contraction of gastrocnemius and soleus, and ankle plantar flexion. A diminished response may indicate herniation of the L5/S1 disc or sciatic nerve palsy. Other causes of reduced reflexes include hypothyroidism.

ANSWER QUESTION 20

1. F – Salter–Harris fracture
2. C – Colles fracture
3. H – None of the above
4. B – Boxer's fracture
5. H – None of the above

These are names for common fractures. The Colles fracture is often caused by a fall on an outstretched hand leading to a distal radius fracture with dorsal angulation. The dinner fork deformity can be seen on plain radiograph. A Smith fracture is also a fracture of the distal radius, but with volar displacement, and occurs due to a fall on an outstretched hand but with a flexed wrist. Salter–Harris fractures are those which involve or relate to a growth plate. This type of fracture requires careful and accurate reduction to ensure further normal growth. A Pott's fracture is only bimalleolar due to eversion of the ankle.

EMQs Paper 4

1. RESPIRATORY

A. Asthma
B. Chronic obstructive pulmonary disease
C. Cystic fibrosis
D. Haemoptysis
E. Pleuritis
F. Pneumonia
G. Pulmonary fibrosis

For each of the following descriptions, select the most appropriate condition. Each option may be used once, more than once or not at all.

1. This condition is associated with a diurnal variation in peak expiratory flow.
2. This condition is associated with an irreversibly reduced forced expiration volume in 1 second (FEV_1):forced vital capacity (FVC) ratio.
3. This condition is associated with impaired mucociliary clearance.
4. This condition is associated with an increased lung compliance.
5. This condition is associated with a reduced vital capacity.

2. ORTHOPAEDICS AND RHEUMATOLOGY

A. Acetylcholine
B. Actin
C. Cardiac muscle
D. Dopamine
E. Fast fibres
F. Myosin
G. Noradrenaline
H. Serotonin
I. Skeletal (striated) muscle
J. Slow fibres
K. Smooth muscle

For each of the following statements concerning muscle fibres, select the correct option. Each option may be used once, more than once or not at all.

1. These fibres appear red because of high levels of myoglobin.
2. This is a neurotransmitter at the neuromuscular junction in skeletal (striated) muscle.

3. This muscle type has slow cycling of actin–myosin cross-bridges.
4. These are thick filaments involved in cross-bridge formation during muscle contraction.
5. Infarction of this muscle type results in characteristic changes on the electrocardiogram.

3. GASTROENTEROLOGY

A. Barrett oesophagus
B. Coeliac disease
C. Cryptosporidiosis
D. Duodenal ulcer
E. Gastric ulcer
F. Hiatus hernia
G. Lymphoma
H. Mucosa-associated lymphoid tissue
 I. Partial villous atrophy
 J. Tropical sprue
K. Whipple disease
L. None of the above

For each of the following scenarios, select the most appropriate diagnosis. Each option may be used once, more than once or not at all.

1. A 69-year-old woman presents with progressive dysphagia. It began with solids but is now preventing the ingestion of liquids. Weight loss has been noted. The patient is a lifelong smoker and drinks approximately 14 units of alcohol a week.
2. A 49-year-old malnourished man presents with abdominal pain, weight loss and arthritis. He also has fatty, offensive stools. A jejunal biopsy shows periodic acid-Schiff positive macrophages.
3. A 61-year-old woman presents with dyspepsia associated with epigastric pain. The pain is worse on eating. She is also suffering from arthritis for which she self medicates with copious non-steroidal anti-inflammatory drugs.
4. An otherwise healthy 43-year-old HIV-positive woman presents following swimming in an inadequately chlorinated pool. She is now suffering from watery diarrhoea, abdominal cramps, vomiting and fever.
5. A 61-year-old man presents with epigastric pain and weight loss. On endoscopy he is found to have a single gastric lesion which is CLO positive.

4. NEUROLOGY

A. Abductor pollicis brevis
B. Adductor pollicis brevis
C. Facial nerve
D. Glossopharyngeal nerve
E. Hypoglossal nerve

F. Lower motor neuron lesion
G. Optic nerve
H. Radial nerve
 I. Trigeminal nerve: mandibular branch
 J. Trigeminal nerve: ophthalmic branch
K. Upper motor neuron lesion

For each of the following questions, select the most appropriate nerve or muscle. Each option may be used once, more than once or not at all.

1. Which structure when damaged results in weakness and wasting of the tongue?
2. Which muscle would be wasted in a median nerve lesion?
3. Which nerve supplies sensation to the cornea?
4. Which type of lesion is associated with diminished or absent reflexes?
5. Which nerve supplies the muscles of facial expression?

5. SPINAL CORD AND SPINAL REFLEXES

A. Corticospinal tract
B. Dorsal column–medial lemniscus
C. Reticulospinal tract
D. Rubrospinal tract
E. Spinothalamic tract
F. Tectospinal tract
G. Vestibulospinal tract
H. None of the above

For each of the following descriptions, select the most appropriate pathway. Each option may be used once, more than once or not at all.

1. This pathway conveys motor information.
2. This pathway conveys temperature information.
3. This pathway conveys light touch information.
4. This pathway conveys pain information.
5. This pathway conveys proprioceptive information.

6. ORTHOPAEDICS AND RHEUMATOLOGY

A. Cancellous bone
B. Cortical bone
C. Hypocalcaemia
D. Osteitis fibrosa cystica
E. Osteogenesis imperfecta
F. Osteomalacia
G. Osteoporosis
H. Paget disease of bone
 I. Periosteum
 J. None of the above

For each of the following descriptions, select the most appropriate type of bone or diagnosis. Each option may be used once, more than once or not at all.

1. This condition is characterized by abnormal type I collagen synthesis.
2. This condition has radiological findings which characteristically include pseudofractures.
3. This condition has a pathognomonic radiological features of a tile-like mosaic with osteoid cement lines.
4. This type of bone makes up to 20% of the human skeleton.
5. This condition is characterized by a decreased bone mineral density.

7. PHARMACOLOGY

  A. Aspirin
  B. Clopidogrel
  C. Low molecular weight heparin
  D. Octaplex
  E. Omeprazole
  F. Ticlopidine
  G. Tirofiban
  H. Unfractionated heparin

A 71-year-old man comes into A & E complaining of chest pain. His ECG shows some inferolateral ischaemic changes with a raised troponin rise. For each of the following descriptions, select the most appropriate drug. Each option may be used once, more than once or not at all.

1. The patient goes for primary percutaneous coronary intervention and has a drug-eluting stent. This drug must be taken for one year.
2. This drug has been shown to interact with clopidogrel.
3. This drug is associated with neutropaenia and thrombotic thrombocyto-paenic purpura.
4. This drug is a glycoprotein IIb/IIIa inhibitor.
5. This drug is an inhibitor of cyclooxygenase.

8. THE CELL

  A. 5p
  B. 7p
  C. 15p
  D. 16p
  E. 17p
  F. 18p
  G. 5q
  H. 7q
  I. 13q
  J. 15q

K. 16q
L. 17q
M. 18q

For each of the following descriptions, select the most appropriate chromosome. Each option may be used once, more than once or not at all.

1. The tumour suppressor gene p53 is located on this chromosome.
2. The tumour suppressor gene RB1 is located on this chromosome.
3. The tumour suppressor gene APC is located on this chromosome.
4. The tumour suppressor gene BRCA1 is located on this chromosome.
5. The tumour suppressor gene NF1 is located on this chromosome.

9. PHYSIOLOGY

A. Acetylcholine deficiency
B. Chemoreceptor trigger zone
C. Dopamine deficiency
D. Excess acetylcholine
E. Excess dopamine
F. Mesolimbic
G. Nigrostriatal
H. Tuberoinfundibular

For each of the following descriptions, select the most appropriate response. Each option may be used once, more than once or not at all.

1. This neurotransmitter problem leads to psychotic symptoms.
2. This pathway is concerned with mood, emotional stability and hallucinations.
3. This pathway is concerned with movement.
4. This pathway is concerned with prolactin secretion.
5. This pathway is concerned with nausea and vomiting.

10. THE CELL

A. Cell membrane
B. Endoplasmic reticulum
C. Golgi apparatus
D. Histones
E. Lysosomes
F. Mitochondria
G. Nucleus
H. Ribosomes

For each of the following statements, select the most appropriate cellular structure. Each option may be used once, more than once or not at all.

1. This structure contains DNA within a double membrane.
2. This structure has an inner membrane folded into cristae.

3. This structure manufactures proteins and is attached to the rough endoplasmic reticulum.
4. This is the semipermeable structure responsible for cellular homeostasis.
5. This structure contains lytic enzymes for the digestion of ingested particles.

11. BIOCHEMISTRY

A. Alanine aminotransferase
B. Creatine kinase
C. Creatinine
D. Gentamicin
E. Oral contraceptive pill
F. Salbutamol
G. Sodium
H. Troponin I
I. Urate
J. Urea
K. Urobilin

For each of the following, select the most appropriate biochemical marker or drug. Each option may be used once, more than once or not at all.

1. Which biochemical marker is elevated following cardiac muscle necrosis?
2. Which biochemical marker is elevated following hepatocyte necrosis?
3. Which biochemical marker is elevated following rhabdomyolysis?
4. Which biochemical marker is elevated in tumour cell lysis after chemotherapy?
5. Which of the above is a cause of renal tubular necrosis?

12. BONE PHYSIOLOGY

A. Bone lining cells
B. Howship lacunae
C. Osteoblasts
D. Osteoclasts
E. Osteocytes
F. Osteoid
G. Osteophyte
H. None of the above

For each of the following descriptions, select the most appropriate term. Each option may be used once, more than once or not at all.

1. An inactive osteoblast.
2. These lie in Howship lacunae.
3. These are responsible for bone production.
4. These are responsible for bone resorption.
5. These may secrete acid phosphatase.

13. GASTROENTEROLOGY

A. Chief cells
B. Chromaffin cells
C. D-cells
D. Enterochromaffin-like cells
E. G-cells
F. Goblet cells
G. Parietal cells
H. None of the above

For each of the following descriptions, select the most appropriate cell group. Each option may be used once, more than once or not at all.

1. These cells produce histamine.
2. These cells secrete gastrin and stimulate enterochromaffin-like cells.
3. These cells produce somatostatin.
4. These cells secrete intrinsic factor.
5. These cells secrete hydrochloric acid.

14. EPITHELIAL AND CONNECTIVE TISSUES

A. Bone morphogenetic protein 4
B. Fibrillin 1
C. Type I collagen
D. Type II collagen
E. Type III collagen
F. Type IV collagen
G. Type V collagen
H. None of the above

For each of the following descriptions, select the most appropriate type of collagen or protein. Each option may be used once, more than once or not at all.

1. This is defective in Stickler syndrome.
2. This is defective in osteogenesis imperfecta.
3. This is defective in Marfan syndrome.
4. This is defective in the vascular subtype of Ehlers–Danlos syndrome.
5. This is defective in the classical subtype of Ehlers–Danlos syndrome.

15. ENDOCRINOLOGY

A. Familial benign hypercalcaemia
B. Malignancy
C. Primary hyperparathyroidism
D. Pseudohypoparathyroidism
E. Pseudopseudohypoparathyroidism
F. Secondary hyperparathyroidism

G. Tertiary hyperparathyroidism

H. None of the above

For each of the following scenarios, select the most appropriate diagnosis. Each option may be used once, more than once or not at all.

1. A patient who had a mastectomy for breast cancer 1 year ago presents with rib pain.
2. A child whose investigations show decreased calcium, increased phosphate and an increased parathyroid hormone (PTH). The child is short, has a round face and his 4th and 5th metacarpals are short.
3. A particularly short child with a round face and short 4th and 5th metacarpals. Bloods for calcium, phosphate and PTH are normal.
4. A patient who presents with kidney stones is found to have a high PTH. Her past medical history includes a pituitary adenoma and a VIPoma. She is known to suffer from multiple endocrine neoplasia type 1 (MEN 1) syndrome.
5. A patient who presents with ureteric colic. His investigations show high calcium and a high PTH. His parathyroids are removed but follow-up blood tests show a persistently high calcium level.

16. GASTROENTEROLOGY

A. Direct inguinal hernia

B. Femoral hernia

C. Incisional hernia

D. Indirect inguinal hernia

E. Paraumbilical hernia

F. Spigelian hernia

G. Umbilical hernia

H. None of the above

For each of the following descriptions, select the most appropriate type of hernia. Each option may be used once, more than once or not at all.

1. A hernia of the aponeurotic layer of the rectus abdominis muscle and semilunar line.
2. The most common type of umbilical hernia.
3. The most common type of inguinal hernia.
4. A hernia involving a strangulated Meckel diverticulum.
5. The most common type of abdominal hernia.

17. ANTIBIOTICS

A. Cefalexin

B. Cefedrolor

C. Cefepime

D. Cefotaxime

E. Ceftioxide

F. Ceftobiprole
G. Cefuroxime
H. None of the above

For each of the following descriptions, select the most appropriate antibiotic. Each option may be used once, more than once or not at all.

1. A fourth-generation cephalosporin.
2. A fifth-generation cephalosporin.
3. A second-generation cephalosporin.
4. A first-generation cephalosporin.
5. A third-generation cephalosporin.

18. ENDOCRINOLOGY

A. Adrenocorticotrophic hormone
B. Empty sella syndrome
C. Growth hormone
D. Kallmann syndrome
E. Pituitary apoplexy
F. Sheehan syndrome
G. Steroids and thyroxine – steroids first
H. Thyroid hormone alone
 I. Steroids and thyroxine – thyroxine first

For each of the following descriptions, select the most appropriate hormone or condition. Each option may be used once, more than once or not at all.

1. This is a rare syndrome, where pituitary infarction ensues after severe postpartum haemorrhage.
2. A patient presents with a poor sense of smell and difficulty differentiating colours.
3. A patient with a known pituitary tumour presents to A & E with severe headache and visual loss.
4. This/these hormone(s) should be replaced on beginning treatment for hypopituitarism.
5. The first hormone(s) to be affected by hypopituitarism.

19. THE CELL

A. Anaphase A
B. Anaphase B
C. Interphase
D. Metaphase
E. Prometaphase
F. Prophase
G. Telophase
H. None of the above

For each of the following descriptions, select the most appropriate stage of the cell cycle. Each option may be used once, more than once or not at all.

1. This is the cell cycle stage where the mitotic spindle is formed.
2. This is the cell cycle stage where chromatin becomes condensed.
3. This is the cell cycle stage where the nuclear envelope reassembles.
4. This is the cell cycle stage where the nuclear membrane breaks down.
5. This is the cell cycle stage where there is an assembly of the contractile ring.

20. GASTROENTEROLOGY

A. Abdominoperineal resection
B. Appendectomy
C. Extended right hemicolectomy
D. Hartmann procedure
E. Lower anterior resection
F. Partial ileal bypass surgery
G. Right hemicolectomy
H. None of the above

For each of the following descriptions, select the most appropriate operation. Each option may be used once, more than once or not at all.

1. This refers to the surgical resection of the rectosigmoid colon with closure of the rectal stump and colostomy formation.
2. This procedure is undertaken for cancer in the proximal two-thirds of the rectum.
3. This procedure is undertaken for cancer in the distal third of the rectum.
4. This refers to the resection of the ascending colon.
5. This procedure is prophylactically performed in patients with ulcerative colitis.

Answers Paper 4

ANSWER QUESTION 1

1. A – Asthma
Asthma is a condition exhibiting airway hypersensitivity and reversible characteristics of obstructive pulmonary disease. As a result, peak expiratory flow readings can vary throughout the day, though readings classically show a morning dip.

2. B – Chronic obstructive pulmonary disease
An irreversible reduction of FEV_1:FVC ratio can be seen in obstructive pulmonary disorders such as chronic obstructive pulmonary disease (COPD). This encompasses chronic bronchitis and emphysema.

3. C – Cystic fibrosis
Cystic fibrosis is a genetic disorder which impairs the function of the secretory glands in the body. The effect is excessive and thick mucus production. The consequence of this in the lung is impaired mucociliary clearance.

4. B – Chronic obstructive pulmonary disease
In COPD the elastic tissue is destroyed and the lung loses some of its natural elastic recoil. This causes a pathological increase in lung compliance.

5. G – Pulmonary fibrosis
Pulmonary fibrosis results in restrictive patterns of lung function secondary to stiffer lungs. In restrictive disorders, all lung volumes and capacities are reduced.

ANSWER QUESTION 2

1. J – Slow fibres
Skeletal (or striated) muscle is composed of fast and slow fibres which are adapted for different functions. Slow fibres are adapted for prolonged muscle contraction (e.g. postural muscles), while fast fibres are used for short-acting, powerful muscle contractions. Slow fibres are also known as red muscle because of their high levels of myoglobin. They have a large number of mitochondria, for high levels of oxidative metabolism. Fast fibres, or white muscle, are larger and have large amounts of glycolytic enzymes for the rapid release of energy.

2. A – Acetylcholine

The motor neuron and muscle fibre form the neuromuscular junction (NMJ). Initiation of a presynaptic action potential results in the influx of calcium ions into the presynaptic cell. Acetylcholine (ACh)-containing vesicles diffuse across the cell and fuse with the neural membrane, releasing ACh into the cleft. Nicotinic ACh receptors on the postsynaptic membrane are activated and result in a positively charged influx (Na^+) into the postsynaptic cell, the end plate potential. If this potential change is above a specific threshold, an action potential is fired. ACh is broken down by acetylcholinesterase in the synaptic cleft and this terminates the response.

3. K – Smooth muscle

Smooth muscle can be divided into two main types: multi-unit, where fibres can contract independently of one another (e.g. ciliary muscle of the iris), and single-unit, whereby muscle fibres contract as a single unit (e.g. visceral muscle of the gut wall). Unlike skeletal muscle, smooth muscle is not organized in a striated fashion, but the myosin filaments are interspersed among the actin filaments. The cycling of cross-bridges between the two filaments is much slower in smooth muscle than skeletal muscle, and this allows for prolonged tonic contraction.

4. F – Myosin

Muscle contraction occurs by cross-bridge formation between thin and thick filaments. Thin filaments are made of actin, while the thick are mainly myosin. Thick and thin filaments are arranged so that they interdigitate with one another. Muscle contraction is brought about by thin filaments moving over the thick filaments via ATP-dependent cross-bridge formation in a 'walk-along' fashion.

5. C – Cardiac muscle

Coronary artery occlusion can result from the rupture of an atherosclerotic plaque and thrombus formation. The area of cardiac muscle that is not being adequately perfused will become ischaemic, and necrosis and infarction can occur. Along with the history, examination and cardiac enzyme tests, the electrocardiogram (ECG) can diagnose a myocardial infarction (MI). Changes in the ECG include elevation of the ST segment, inversion of T waves and the presence of pathological Q waves. The leads affected by these changes indicate the area of the infarcted myocardium and the vessel that is occluded, as shown in the table below.

ECG leads	Location of infarct	Vessel affected
II, III, aVF	Inferior MI	Right coronary artery
V2–5	Anterior MI	Left main coronary artery
I, aVL, V3–6	Anterolateral MI	Left anterior descending (LAD) artery
V1–3	Anteroseptal MI	Circumflex or diagonal branch of the LAD
Reciprocal changes in V1–4	Posterior MI	Left circumflex or right coronary artery

ANSWER QUESTION 3

1. L – None of the above
2. K – Whipple disease
3. E – Gastric ulcer
4. C – Cryptosporidiosis
5. E – Gastric ulcer

Whipple disease is a rare systemic infection caused by the bacterium *Tropheryma whipplei*. It may affect any part of the body but is most commonly considered a gastrointestinal disease. Biopsy will reveal periodic acid-Schiff (PAS)-positive macrophage inclusions. Treatment is with antibiotics for up to 2 years, and this may not be successful and result in relapse. Cryptosporidiosis is a parasitic disease which will cause self-limiting diarrhoea in those not immunocompromised. However, in the immunocompromised a more severe form may manifest.

ANSWER QUESTION 4

1. E – Hypoglossal nerve

Upon denervation a muscle will become wasted and atrophic. The hypoglossal nerve (cranial nerve XII) is a motor nerve that supplies the tongue, and so ipsilateral wasting may be evident with hypoglossal nerve lesions. Deviation on protrusion towards the affected side is a localizing feature. Motor neuron disease with bulbar involvement is one such cause.

2. A – Abductor pollicis brevis

The median nerve supplies the muscles of the thenar eminence: abductor pollicis brevis, flexor pollicis brevis and opponens pollicis. Median nerve damage (e.g. carpal tunnel syndrome) leads to wasting of the thenar eminence and weak movements of the thumb. Loss of sensation to the lateral three-and-a-half digits also occurs.

3. J – Trigeminal nerve: ophthalmic branch

The trigeminal nerve (cranial nerve V) has three components: ophthalmic, maxillary and mandibular. Its motor component supplies the muscles of mastication, which include the temporalis, masseter and pterygoids. The ophthalmic branch supplies sensation to the cornea and thus is the afferent neuron in the corneal reflex.

4. F – Lower motor neuron lesion

Lower motor neuron lesions occur when there is nerve damage between the anterior horn cell (or cranial nerve nuclei) and the motor end-plate. An upper motor neuron lesion occurs anywhere proximal to this point. The differences in symptoms and signs guide the diagnosis. The main differences are as given in the table below.

	Upper motor neuron	Lower motor neuron
Power	Weakness	Weakness
Reflexes	Hyperreflexia	Absent/diminished
	Positive Babinski reflex	
Tone	Increased tone	Decreased tone
Wasting	Only if chronic	Yes
Fasciculation	No	Yes

5. C – Facial nerve

As the name suggests, the facial nerve (cranial nerve VII) supplies the muscles of facial expression. It also supplies taste to the anterior two-thirds of the tongue and motor function to stapedius in the middle ear. The differences between upper and lower motor neuron lesions are important when assessing facial nerve palsy. In a lower motor neuron lesion (e.g. Bell's palsy), the whole ipsilateral side of the face is affected, with weakness throughout. However, the frontalis muscle of the forehead is spared in an upper motor neuron lesion (e.g. following a stroke).

ANSWER QUESTION 5

1. A – Corticospinal tract
2. E – Spinothalamic tract
3. B – Dorsal column–medial lemniscus
4. E – Spinothalamic tract
5. B – Dorsal column–medial lemniscus

The dorsal column–medial lemniscus pathway transmits fine touch, vibration and proprioceptive information. The spinothalamic tract transmits information about pain, temperature, itch and crude touch. The corticospinal tract is concerned specifically with discrete voluntary skilled movements, especially of the distal parts of the limbs. The lateral vestibulospinal tract coordinates extensor muscle tone and equilibrium in response to gravity. The medial vestibulospinal tract coordinates head and neck position. The tectospinal tract coordinates head and eye movements. It mediates reflex postural movements of the head in response to visual and auditory stimuli through a connection between the midbrain tectum and the spinal cord.

ANSWER QUESTION 6

1. E – Osteogenesis imperfecta
2. F – Osteomalacia
3. H – Paget disease of bone
4. A – Cancellous bone
5. G – Osteoporosis

Osteogenesis imperfecta is a genetic disorder of variable inheritance pattern which involves a deficiency in type I collagen. Affected patients have bones that fracture easily, loose joints and poor muscle tone. Osteomalacia is a disorder of bone mineralization and is characteristically associated with the presence of pseudofractures (or Looser zones) on radiology. These appear as horizontal lucencies that only travel partway across a bone and are commonly seen in the public rami and proximal femurs. In children, osteomalacia is known as rickets. A common cause for this is vitamin D deficiency. Paget disease of the bone is a chronic disease of bone turnover which is divided into three stages: osteolytic, osteolytic–osteosclerotic and quiescent osteosclerotic. Fifteen percent involves just one bone and there is a predilection to the cranial bones and spine. The patient may suffer from pain, microfractures and nerve compression. Note the screening test result will be a markedly raised alkaline phosphatase. Cancellous bone includes the vertebrae and pelvis, and this type of bone comprises approximately 20% of the skeleton. Cancellous bone is far more metabolically active than cortical bone. Cancellous bone lamellae do not form Haversian systems.

ANSWER QUESTION 7

1. B – Clopidogrel
Clopidogrel is an extremely important drug to cardiologists. Prior to the use of clopidogrel, a drug called ticlopidine was used. This drug was no longer used when clopidogrel hit the market, as ticlopidine was found to be associated with neutropaenia and thrombotic thrombocytopaenic purpura (TTP). Any patient who has a drug-eluting stent must remain on clopidogrel for 1 year, and those with a bare metal stent require 1 month's treatment with clopidogrel. Stents become endothelialized, and after this point the high risk of clot formation within the stent is significantly reduced. This endothelialization process takes longer with drug-eluting stents, and therefore cover with clopidogrel is needed for a longer period of time.

2. E – Omeprazole
There is a potentially serious drug interaction between proton pump inhibitors (such as omeprazole and lansoprazole) and clopidogrel. The interaction is thought to involve the P450 cytochrome family. Many cardiologists are therefore changing their patients from proton pump inhibitors to the more 'old-fashioned' histamine H_2-receptor antagonists, such as ranitidine, due to the decreased efficacy of clopidogrel.

3. F – Ticlopidine
Ticlopidine was the drug used before clopidogrel was available. It was found to have the adverse side-effects of neutropaenia and TTP, which is a disorder of blood coagulation resulting in extensive microscopic small vessel thrombosis. Patients present with microangiopathic haemolytic anaemia, thrombocytopaenia, renal failure, fevers and bizarre neurological symptoms.

4. G – Tirofiban

Tirofiban is a glycoprotein IIb/IIIa inhibitor which inhibits platelet aggregation and thrombus formation. It is licensed in the treatment of unstable angina and non-ST elevation myocardial infarction. It is commonly used in patients who are likely to subsequently go for percutaneous transluminal coronary angioplasty. Tirofiban has been associated with an approximate 1.4% risk of major bleeding and just over 10% risk of minor bleeding.

5. A – Aspirin

Aspirin is a particularly important drug in the prevention and treatment of cardiovascular disease. It works by the inhibition of cyclooxygenase with subsequent inhibition of the production of thromboxane A_2, which is important in the activation of platelet aggregation.

ANSWER QUESTION 8

1. E – 17p
The p53 tumour suppressor gene, which is implicated in more than 50% of all cancers, is located on chromosome 17p.

2. I – 13q
The RB1 gene is implicated in causing the rare eye cancer retinoblastoma. The RB1 gene can be found on chromosome 13q.

3. G – 5q
The tumour suppressor gene APC is located on chromosome 5q.

4. L – 17q
BRCA1 is a tumour suppressor gene which has been implicated in breast and ovarian cancer. It is located on chromosome 17q.

5. L – 17q
NF1 is a tumour suppressor gene which has been implicated in neurofibrosarcoma. It is located on chromosome 17q.

ANSWER QUESTION 9

1. E – Excess dopamine
There are many hypotheses of the pathogenesis of schizophrenia. The effect of dopamine antagonists as antipsychotics supports the hypothesis of excess dopamine transmission in schizophrenia.

2. F – Mesolimbic
The mesolimbic pathway is involved with delusions, hallucinations and drug dependence. It also plays a role in the pleasurable effects of food, sex and drugs of abuse.

3. G – Nigrostriatal
The nigrostriatal pathway is involved with controlling movement. Antagonism in this area leads to clinical signs of parkinsonism, and a lack of dopamine in this area causes Parkinson disease.

4. H – Tuberoinfundibular
Dopamine released by neurones in the tuberoinfundibular pathway acts via D2 receptors to inhibit prolactin secretion. For this reason bromocriptine, a dopamine receptor agonist, is used in the treatment of galactorrhoea. Conversely, antipsychotics which block D2 can lead to breast swelling, pain and lactation.

5. B – Chemoreceptor trigger zone
Antagonism of dopamine receptors in this area prevents nausea and vomiting. This is the mechanism of action of the antiemetic domperidone, which is particularly useful in the control of nausea associated with cytotoxic drugs.

ANSWER QUESTION 10

1. G – Nucleus
The nucleus houses the chromosomes which contain the genetic material and instructions for growth and function. The nuclear membrane has pores that allow the transfer of molecules in and out of the cell. The central nucleoli contain RNA and protein, which are involved in ribosomal production.

2. F – Mitochondria
The mitochondria are responsible for generating ATP, which is the cell's energy source, via oxidative phosphorylation. The inner membrane is folded into cristae which increase the surface area for the electron transport chain to occur. The Krebs cycle also occurs in the mitochondria.

3. H – Ribosomes
Ribosomes are responsible for translation and thus protein synthesis. They are attached along the endoplasmic reticulum. Protein modification and processing occurs in the lumen of the rough endoplasmic reticulum, while smooth endoplasmic reticulum contains the P450 cytochrome enzymes, which are involved in detoxification and metabolism.

4. A – Cell membrane
The cell membrane controls the transport of solute in and out of the cell, via specialized transport mechanisms. Transporters vary depending on the needs and function of the cell. For example, cells along the renal tubule are specialized with different transporters to allow filtration and reabsorption of the necessary solutes.

5. E – Lysosomes

Lysosomes are involved in the digestion of ingested macromolecules. They contain lytic enzymes, which cause destruction if they pathologically leak. For example, in cellular necrosis, cell lysis results in the release of lytic enzymes that furthers tissue damage.

ANSWER QUESTION 11

1. H – Troponin I

Troponin I is elevated after myocardial infarction (MI) and should be tested for 12 hours after the onset of symptoms. Along with the history and electrocardiogram (ECG) findings, cardiac enzymes are used to make the diagnosis of an acute coronary syndrome (ACS). ACS consists of three conditions: ST-elevation MI (STEMI), non-ST-elevation MI (NSTEMI) and unstable angina. Most hospitals have an ACS protocol, which should be followed when managing these patients. It involves giving oxygen, relieving pain, nitrates (usually glyceryl trinitrate [GTN] spray), aspirin and an anti-platelet agent. ACE inhibitors, statins and β-blockers may also be started.

2. A – Alanine aminotransferase

Hepatocellular necrosis occurs in acute liver failure. Causes include toxins (e.g. paracetamol overdose or alcohol), hepatitis virus or metabolic causes such as haemochromatosis. Markers of intrinsic liver function, such as alanine aminotransferase (ALT) and aspartate aminotransferase (AST), will be markedly elevated. The transaminases can be used to detect hepatocyte damage, while γ-glutamyltransferase (GGT) and alkaline phosphatase (ALP) are more useful markers of obstruction.

3. B – Creatine kinase

Rhabdomyolysis is the breakdown of skeletal muscle, which may be caused by inactivity, crush injury or toxins (e.g. MDMA). The breakdown products of muscle include myoglobin, which can accumulate and cause tubular damage. Myoglobin is excreted by the kidney and causes the urine to become slightly brown in colour. Creatine kinase levels are also high. This is a common phenomenon in elderly patients who are found on the floor after a fall.

4. I – Urate

Tumour lysis syndrome can occur after breakdown of a tumour following chemotherapy, resulting in the release of uric acid. The cancers most frequently associated with tumour lysis syndrome are leukaemias and lymphomas. Hyperkalaemia can result in arrhythmias, and hyperuricaemia can result in renal failure. Other features include hyperphosphataemia and hypocalcaemia. Adequate hydration and allopurinol can reduce the risk of tumour lysis syndrome.

5. D – Gentamicin

Gentamicin can cause acute tubular necrosis. Levels should be monitored to avoid nephrotoxicity, and the once-a-day high-dose regimen should be avoided in patients with a low creatinine clearance. Gentamicin is excreted primarily by the kidney and thus levels can accumulate when renal function is poor. Other adverse effects include ototoxicity and hearing loss, antibiotic-associated colitis and stomatitis.

ANSWER QUESTION 12

1. A – Bone lining cells
2. D – Osteoclasts
3. C – Osteoblasts
4. D – Osteoclasts
5. D – Osteoclasts

Osteoblasts produce osteoid which when mineralized becomes bone. Osteoclasts are the cells which resorb bone. They lie in Howship lacunae, which are produced through the breakdown of the bone surface. Osteophytes are otherwise known as bone spurs and occur in arthritides. Bone lining cells are inactive osteoblasts and act as a barrier.

ANSWER QUESTION 13

1. D – Enterochromaffin-like cells
2. E – G-cells
3. C – D-cells
4. G – Parietal cells
5. G – Parietal cells

Histamine is produced and secreted by enterochromaffin cells. They are found in the gastric mucosa close to parietal cells. Production is stimulated by gastrin, which is secreted by the G-cells in the gastric epithelium. Histamine and gastrin work synergistically to stimulate the production of hydrochloric acid from parietal cells. Somatostatin is produced by the D-cells. Parietal cells produce gastric acid in response to histamine, acetylcholine and gastrin. The cells themselves contain canaliculi from which gastric acid is secreted by active transport into the stomach. Goblet cells are the second most common epithelial cell type in the gastrointestinal tract. They increase in number along the length of the intestine. They contain mucous granules which accumulate at the apical (luminal) end of the cell, thus giving the cell a goblet-shaped appearance. The mucus secreted facilitates the passage of material through the bowel.

ANSWER QUESTION 14

1. D – Type II collagen
2. C – Type I collagen

3. B – Fibrillin 1
4. E – Type III collagen
5. G – Type V collagen

Stickler syndrome is caused by defects in the COL11A1 and COL11A2 genes leading to defective type II and XI collagen production. This leads to eye abnormalities, hearing loss and arthritis. Ehlers–Danlos syndrome (EDS) is a group of disorders in which there is defective collagen synthesis. In the most common form there is a mutation of the vascular EDS and tenascin-X genes. In classical EDS there is a genetic defect which causes defective type V and I collagen. There is also a vascularly aggressive type where there is a defect in type III collagen.

Marfan syndrome is caused by a mutation of the FBN1 (fibrillin 1) gene which is necessary for the production of fibrillin – a component required for the correct formation of the extracellular matrix which includes the production and maintenance of elastic fibres. The aortic ligaments and the ciliary muscles are most affected.

Osteogenesis imperfecta (OI) patients suffer from an inability to make well-functioning connective tissue, or are born with defective connective tissue. OI usually defined by a deficiency in type I collagen. The substitution of glycine to larger amino acids within the collagen triple helix structure leads to an abnormal structure which should be hydrolysed by the body. If it is not, the relationship between the collagen and mineralization is altered, leading to brittleness.

Fibrodysplasia ossificans progressiva (FOP) is a rare mutation of the repair mechanism of fibrous tissue where tissue becomes ossified when damaged. Pseudoxanthoma elasticum causes fragmentation and mineralization of elastic fibres in the skin, eyes and blood vessels. About 80% of cases have a detectable mutation of the *ABCC5* gene.

ANSWER QUESTION 15

1. B – Malignancy
2. D – Pseudohypoparathyroidism
3. E – Pseudopseudohypoparathyroidism
4. G – Tertiary hyperparathyroidism
5. A – Familial benign hypercalcaemia

Patients with pseudohypoparathyroidism are resistant to PTH, leading to low calcium and high phosphate with an inappropriately high PTH. Pseudopseudohypoparathyroidism patients are born phenotypically similar to those with pseudohypoparathyroidism but are biochemically normal. Tertiary hyperparathyroidism is a state of excessive PTH secretion after a prolonged period of secondary hyperparathyroidism.

ANSWER QUESTION 16

1. F – Spigelian hernia
2. E – Paraumbilical hernia
3. D – Indirect inguinal hernia
4. H – None of the above
5. D – Indirect inguinal hernia

A Spigelian hernia is a hernia of the aponeurotic layer of the rectus abdominis muscle and the semilunar line. The defect associated with a Speglian hernia is often quite small and consequently the hernias are at increased risk of strangulation. Inguinal hernias are the most common type of abdominal hernia, and of these, indirect hernias occur most frequently. A hernia involving a strangulated Meckel diverticulum is also known as a Littré hernia and can result in a small bowel fistula.

ANSWER QUESTION 17

1. C – Cefepime
2. F – Ceftobiprole
3. G – Cefuroxime
4. A – Cefalexin
5. D – Cefotaxime

First-generation cephalosporins are moderate spectrum agents. Second-generation cephalosporins have greater action against Gram-negative organisms and are more resistant to beta-lactamase. Third-generation cephalosporins are able to penetrate the central nervous system. Fourth-generation cephalosporins have greater resistance to beta-lactamase than the third generation. They are used in meningitis and pseudomonas. Fifth-generation cephalosporins are a new type of drug which are effective against pseudomonas.

ANSWER QUESTION 18

1. F – Sheehan syndrome
Sheehan syndrome, or postpartum pituitary necrosis, is a rare complication of postpartum haemorrhage. The anterior pituitary enlarges during pregnancy in preparation for lactation. However, the blood supply does not mirror the increase. Major postpartum haemorrhage and hypotension can therefore lead to ischaemia of the pituitary gland.

2. D – Kallmann syndrome
Kallmann syndrome describes a genetic GnRH (gonadotrophin-releasing hormone) deficiency which results in hypogonadism. Patients also suffer with anosmia and it can be associated with kidney abnormalities and midline facial deformities.

3. E – Pituitary apoplexy
Pituitary apoplexy occurs when there is infarction or haemorrhage of the pituitary. It may be life-threatening and needs urgent surgical review.

4. G – Steroids and thyroxine – steroids first
Both thyroxine and steroids are required, but giving thyroxine before steroids can precipitate an adrenal crisis.

5. C – Growth hormone
Growth hormone (GH) is the first hormone to be affected by hypopituitarism, and so GH levels are certain to be abnormal if all other pituitary tests are deranged (panhypopituitarism). The most common cause of hypopituitarism is a tumour, and treatment involves correcting the deranged hormone levels, treating the cause and managing the complications.

ANSWER QUESTION 19

1. F – Prophase
2. F – Prophase
3. G – Telophase
4. E – Prometaphase
5. G – Telophase

During prophase the replicated chromosomes condense and the duplicated centrosomes migrate to the opposite sides of the nucleus and begin the assembly of the spindle microtubules. The mitotic spindle forms outside the nucleus between the two centrosomes. Each of the condensed chromosomes consists of two sister chromatids which have a kinetochore each. The microtubules are in a dynamic state and allow the radial microtubules to form around each centrosome and consequently form poles.

During prometaphase the nuclear membrane breaks down and the chromosomes are attached to the spindle via the kinetochore at the centromere region of the chromosome. In late prometaphase the microtubule from the opposite pole is captured by the sister kinetochore and the chromosome slides rapidly towards the centre along the microtubules. Metaphase occurs when the chromosomes are aligned at the equator of the spindle. The mitotic checkpoint is active from the start of prometaphase until the end of metaphase. It senses the completion of chromosome alignment and it is after this has occurred that anaphase may commence.

During anaphase the paired chromatids separate to form the two daughter chromosomes. It is here that cohesin holds the sister chromatids together. During anaphase A the cohesin is broken down and the microtubules become shorter, and the daughter chromosomes are pulled towards opposite spindle poles. In anaphase B the centrosomes migrate apart. Telophase is marked by the arrival of the daughter chromosomes at the poles. The nuclear envelope reassembles at each pole and the contractile ring assembles for the start of cytokinesis.

ANSWER QUESTION 20

1. D – Hartmann procedure
2. E – Lower anterior resection
3. A – Abdominoperineal resection
4. G – Right hemicolectomy
5. H – None of the above

An abdominoperineal (AP) resection is performed when a tumour lies low in the rectum and cannot be removed without loss or damage to the anus. This is in comparison to a lower anterior resection, where the anus will be preserved. A Hartmann procedure is performed in emergency situations where immediate anastomosis is impossible. It is hoped the colostomy will be reversed, but this only occurs in up to one-third of patients. A panproctocolectomy may be performed in a patient with ulcerative colitis as this is curative.

EMQs Paper 5

1. GASTROENTEROLOGY

A. Bannayan–Riley–Ruvalcaba syndrome
B. Cowden syndrome
C. Familial adenomatous polyposis
D. Gardner syndrome
E. Hereditary nonpolyposis colorectal cancer
F. Juvenile polyposis syndrome
G. Peutz–Jeghers syndrome
H. Turcot syndrome
I. None of the above

For each of the following scenarios, select the most appropriate condition. Each option may be used once, more than once or not at all.

1. A 40-year-old man presents with a 3-month history of fatigue, constipation, tenesmus and weight loss. Several small growths which are hard and bony on palpation are noticeable on his head and jaw line.
2. A 40-year-old woman presents with a 2-month history of malaise, weight loss and constipation and a recent episode of rectal bleeding 2 days ago. She has a noticeable goitre, which is found to be multinodular on examination.
3. A 50-year-old woman with a past history of endometrial cancer is recently diagnosed with colorectal cancer. Genetic testing shows a mutation in the *MLH1* gene.
4. A 20-year-old man presents with a 4-month history of worsening constipation and occasional rectal bleeding. Colonoscopy shows numerous polyps, and genetic testing reveals a mutation in the APC gene. His father and paternal grandfather both died of colorectal cancer before the age of 50.
5. A 15-year-old boy presents with a 2-week history of abdominal pain and rectal bleeding. Colonoscopy reveals multiple polyps throughout the colon and a biopsy further reveals cellular overgrowth along with elongated, frond-like epithelium and a cystic dilation of glands. He also has distinct perioral pigmentation.

2. URINARY SYSTEM: ANATOMY AND PHYSIOLOGY

A. Diabetes insipidus
B. Diabetes mellitus

C. Doxazosin use
D. Finasteride use
E. Furosemide use
F. Recent arterial blood gas sampling
G. Recent catheterization
H. Recent venepuncture
I. Spironolactone use
J. Syndrome of inappropriate antidiuretic hormone secretion (SIADH)

For each of the following biochemical findings, select the single most likely cause. Each option may be used once, more than once or not at all. Note, normal values are: Na$^+$ 137–145 mmol/L, K$^+$ 3.6–5.8 mmol/L, prostate specific antigen (PSA) < 4 ng/mL.

1. Na$^+$ = 121 mmol/L
2. K$^+$ = 6.5 mmol/L
3. Na$^+$ = 150 mmol/L
4. K$^+$ = 2.8 mmol/L
5. PSA = 10 ng/mL

3. GASTROENTEROLOGY

A. Antiepidermal transglutaminase
B. Antigliadin antibodies
C. Antimicrosomal antibodies
D. Antimitochondrial antibodies
E. Antireticulin antibodies
F. Anti-tissue transglutaminase antibodies
G. Anti-topoisomerase antibodies
H. None of the above

For each of the following descriptions, select the most appropriate antibody. Each option may be used once, more than once or not at all.

1. The most specific and sensitive antibody for coeliac disease in adults.
2. The most specific and sensitive antibody for coeliac disease in children under the age of 5.
3. These IgG antibodies may be raised in a patient with coeliac disease.
4. This may be raised in a patient with systemic sclerosis.
5. An antibody associated with dermatitis herpetiformis.

4. ORTHOPAEDICS AND RHEUMATOLOGY

A. Addison disease
B. Alopecia
C. Graves disease
D. Motor neuron disease
E. Multiple sclerosis
F. Myasthenia gravis

G. Pernicious anaemia
H. Rheumatoid arthritis
 I. Systemic lupus erythematosus
 J. Type I diabetes mellitus
K. Type II diabetes mellitus
 L. Vitiligo

Inefficient apoptosis can result in the development of auto-antibodies and autoimmune conditions. For each of the following, select the most appropriate autoimmune condition. Each option may be used once, more than once or not at all.

1. Which autoimmune condition is caused by autoantibodies against thyroid-stimulating hormone receptors?
2. Which autoimmune condition is characterized by multisystem involvement and anti–double-stranded DNA antibodies?
3. Which autoimmune condition is characterized by the destruction of pancreatic β-islet cells?
4. Which autoimmune condition is caused by auto-antibodies against intrinsic factor?
5. Which autoimmune condition results in decreased transmission at the neuromuscular junction?

5. CARDIOLOGY

A. Anterolateral myocardial infarction
B. Anterior ST-elevation myocardial infarction
C. Aorta
D. Inferior non–ST-elevation myocardial infarction
E. Inferior ST-elevation myocardial infarction
 F. Internal carotid artery
G. Left anterior descending artery
H. Posterior myocardial infarction
 I. Right coronary artery
 J. Septal myocardial infarction
K. Stable angina
 L. Unstable angina

For each of the following questions concerning cardiac muscle infarction, select the most appropriate option. Each option may be used once, more than once or not at all.

1. Which vessel is occluded if there is infarction of the inferior myocardium?
2. What type of myocardial infarction can be diagnosed from ST elevation and Q wave formation in leads V3–6, I and aVL on the electrocardiogram?
3. What type of infarction can be diagnosed from ST segment elevation in the 'chest leads'?

4. What condition would be diagnosed with chest pain only evident on exertion?
5. What type of infarction is diagnosed from ST depression in leads V1–3, and a prominent R wave in V1?

6. NEUROLOGY

A. Alzheimer disease
B. Creutzfeldt–Jakob disease
C. Delirium
D. Huntington disease
E. Lambert–Eaton syndrome
F. Motor neuron disease
G. Multiple sclerosis
H. Parkinson disease
I. Parkinsonism
J. Schizophrenia
K. Subacute combined degeneration of the cord

Apoptosis and necrosis are involved in the pathogenesis of neurodegenerative disorders. For each of the following questions, select the correct condition. Each option may be used once, more than once or not at all.

1. Which neurodegenerative disorder is characterized by neurofibrillary tangles?
2. Which neurodegenerative disorder is characterized by Lewy bodies?
3. Which neurodegenerative disorder results from γ-aminobutyric acid (GABA)-ergic cell death in the striatum?
4. Which neurodegenerative disorder results in degeneration of motor neurones?
5. Which neurodegenerative disorder results from the accumulation of prion proteins?

7. STRUCTURE OF EPITHELIAL AND CONNECTIVE TISSUES

A. Columnar epithelium
B. Cuboidal epithelium
C. Keratinized epithelium
D. Pseudostratified epithelium
E. Squamous epithelium
F. Transitional epithelium
G. All of the above
H. None of the above

For each of the following descriptions, select the most appropriate type of epithelium. Each option may be used once, more than once or not at all.

1. This epithelium often has oval cell nuclei which are arranged in rows.
2. This epithelium is often arranged in an oval pattern.

3. This epithelium, when viewed superiorly, appears to fit together like a tiled floor.
4. This epithelium, when viewed laterally, shows the cells are stacked in tightly packed layers.
5. This epithelium often has oval cell nuclei arranged at different levels within cells.

8. RESPIRATORY

A. Alveolar pressure
B. Alveolar pressure = transmural pressure
C. Intrapleural pressure = atmospheric pressure
D. Negative alveolar pressure
E. Negative intrapleural pressure
F. Positive intrapleural pressure
G. Transmural pressure
H. Transmural pressure = atmospheric pressure

For each of the following descriptions, select the most appropriate response. Each option may be used once, more than once or not at all.

1. The pressure in the space between the parietal and visceral linings during forceful expiration.
2. The pressure in the space between the parietal and visceral linings during normal inspiration.
3. The pressure difference across the walls of the lung.
4. This state causes lung collapse.
5. This pressure is zero at rest.

9. GASTROENTEROLOGY

A. Acute appendicitis
B. Carcinoma of the sigmoid colon
C. Coeliac disease
D. Crohn disease
E. Diverticular disease
F. Hirschsprung disease
G. Hyperplastic polyp
H. Pseudomembranous colitis
I. Ulcerative colitis
J. None of the above

For each of the following colonoscopy findings, select the most appropriate diagnosis. Each option may be used once, more than once or not at all.

1. Colonoscopy reveals several outpouchings into the mucosa extruding through the muscle.

2. Colonoscopy reveals a membrane-like material covering the epithelium. Biopsy reveals this is comprised of mucin, fibrin, polymorphs and leukocyte and epithelial debris.

3. Colonoscopy reveals a large mass in the sigmoid colon. Biopsy reveals a neoplasm with multiple blood vessels categorized as an adenocarcinoma.

4. Colonoscopy reveals an oedematous reddened colon. Biopsy reveals a continuous superficial ulceration of the colon.

5. Colonoscopy reveals an oedematous, reddened terminal ileum. Biopsy uncovers transmural inflammation with the presence of granulomas.

10. PHARMACOLOGY

A. Atenolol
B. Candesartan
C. Digoxin
D. Doxazosin
E. Lignocaine
F. Nicorandil
G. Nifedipine
H. Nitroprusside

For each of the following descriptions, select the most appropriate vasodilator drug. Each option may be used once, more than once or not at all.

1. This drug is a calcium antagonist.
2. This drug acts via nitric oxide release.
3. This drug is a potassium channel activator.
4. This drug is an inhibitor of sympathetic vasoconstriction.
5. This drug is an angiotensin II receptor antagonist.

11. ENDOCRINOLOGY

A. Adrenal carcinoma
B. Adrenalectomy
C. Bilateral adrenocortical hyperplasia
D. Dexamethasone
E. Eplerenone
F. Ramipril
G. Renal artery stenosis
H. Spironolactone

For each of the following descriptions, select the most appropriate drug or condition. Each option may be used once, more than once or not at all.

1. This is the treatment for Conn's syndrome.
2. This is used given before definite treatment in Conn's syndrome.

3. This is the treatment for glucocorticoid remediable aldosteronism.
4. This is a newer treatment for adrenal hyperplasia.
5. This is a cause of secondary hyperaldosteronism.

12. CARDIOLOGY

A. Atrial fibrillation
B. Cardiac tamponade
C. Complete heart block
D. Dressler syndrome
E. Left ventricular failure
F. Mitral regurgitation
G. Right ventricular failure
H. Ventricular tachycardia

For each of the following scenarios, select the most appropriate complication post-myocardial infarction (MI). Each option may be used once, more than once or not at all.

1. A patient had an ST elevation in leads V1–V5 and was treated with primary percutaneous coronary intervention for an ST elevation MI. His troponin was 33.97. His electrocardiogram (ECG) now shows a ventricular rate of 40 beats per minute, and P-waves at a rate of 90 beats per minute, which seem to 'march through' the trace.
2. A patient returns to clinic for follow up after sustaining an MI 4 weeks ago. She complains of chest pains which improve on leaning forwards and some fevers. Chest X-ray reveals pleural effusions, and her full blood count reveals a haemoglobin of 9.8 g/dL.
3. A female patient suffered a non-ST elevation MI 1 week ago. She has progressively become short of breath on exertion and has a few bibasal crackles. Jugular venous pressure is not elevated.
4. A patient is reviewed in clinic 6 weeks after suffering an MI. His routine ECG shows no P-waves, and the ventricular rate seems to be irregular.
5. A patient has suffered an MI and is currently in accident and emergency. She suddenly drops her blood pressure and becomes extremely confused. The monitor shows a regular broad QRS complex pattern.

13. RESPIRATORY

A. Ethmoid air cells
B. Frontal sinus
C. Mastoid cells
D. Maxillary and ethmoid sinuses
E. Maxillary sinus
F. Sphenoid sinus
G. All of the above
H. None of the above

For each of the following descriptions, select the most appropriate sinus or cell group. Each option may be used once, more than once or not at all.

1. These are paranasal sinuses that do not arise from outpouchings of the nasal cavity.
2. These are the most variable in location and structure.
3. This contains the highest density of goblet cells.
4. This is supplied by the supraorbital nerve.
5. This can develop a cholesteatoma.

14. ORTHOPAEDICS AND RHEUMATOLOGY

A. Axillary nerve
B. Femoral nerve
C. Lateral cutaneous nerve
D. Median nerve
E. Musculocutaneous nerve
F. Obturator nerve
G. Radial nerve
H. Sciatic nerve
I. Spinal accessory nerve
J. Ulnar nerve

For each of the following, select the correct nerve in question. Each option may be used once, more than once or not at all.

1. Which nerve is vulnerable to damage in anterior shoulder dislocation?
2. Which nerve is vulnerable to damage in posterior hip dislocation?
3. Which nerve is vulnerable to damage in humeral shaft fracture?
4. Which nerve of the hand is vulnerable to damage in acromegaly?
5. Which nerve is vulnerable to compression as it passes under the inguinal ligament and is associated with weight change (increase or decrease)?

15. GASTROENTEROLOGY

A. Angular cheilitis
B. Aphthous ulcer
C. Erythroplakia
D. Glossitis
E. Hairy leukoplakia
F. Koilonychia
G. Leukonychia
H. Leukoplakia
I. None of the above

For each of the following descriptions, select the most appropriate condition. Each option may be used once, more than once or not at all.

1. This is always associated with iron deficiency anaemia.
2. This is associated with squamous cell carcinoma.

3. This is associated with pernicious anaemia.
4. This can be associated with oesophageal carcinoma.
5. This is associated with human immunodeficiency virus infection.

EMQs Paper 5

16. URINARY SYSTEM
A. Benign prostatic hyperplasia
B. Cystitis
C. Detrusor instability
D. Haemorrhage
E. Polycystic kidney disease
F. Pyelonephritis
G. Renal artery stenosis
H. Renal calculi
 I. Renal cell carcinoma
 J. Tubular necrosis

For each of the following statements, select the single most likely cause. Each option may be used once, more than once or not at all.

1. This is a cause of pre-renal failure.
2. This is a cause of post-renal failure in women.
3. This is an inherited predisposition to subarachnoid haemorrhage.
4. This is a cause of 'cannon-ball' lesions on chest X ray.
5. This is a cause of renal impairment following gentamicin therapy.

17. ENDOCRINOLOGY
A. Anxiety
B. Fluid resuscitation
C. Hydrocortisone IV
D. Hydrocortisone PO
E. Hyperglycaemia
F. Hyperpigmentation of palmar creases
G. Hypoglycaemia
H. Hypopigmentation of palmar creases
 I. Surgery

For each of the following descriptions, select the most appropriate response. Each option may be used once, more than once or not at all.

1. Addisonian crisis may be precipitated by this.
2. This is the result of a blood glucose test during an Addisonian crisis.
3. This is the initial management of an Addisonian crisis.
4. This is given as an additional treatment in the acute phase of an Addisonian crisis.
5. This may be seen on examination in patient with adrenal insufficiency.

111

18. NEUROLOGY

A. Corticospinal tract
B. Raphespinal tract
C. Reticulospinal tract
D. Spinocerebellar tract
E. Spinothalamic tract
F. Tectospinal tract
G. Vestibulospinal tract
H. None of the above

For each of the following descriptions, select the most appropriate spinal tract. Each option may be used once, more than once or not at all.

1. This controls locomotion and postural control.
2. This controls maintenance of a centre of gravity between the feet.
3. This controls modulation of sensory transmission.
4. This is thought to control head and trunk orientation following visual and auditory stimuli.
5. This conveys information to the cerebellum about limb and joint position.

19. THE CELL

A. A-bands
B. Actin
C. Actinin
D. Calcium
E. I-bands
F. Myosin
G. Tropomyosin
H. Troponin
I. Z-lines

For each of the following descriptions, select the most appropriate response. Each option may be used once, more than once or not at all.

1. The interval between these is defined as a sarcomere.
2. Thin myofilaments consist mainly of this.
3. Thick myofilaments consist mainly of this.
4. Z-lines contain this protein.
5. The I-band consists of this.

20. GASTROENTEROLOGY

A. Carman meniscus sign
B. Irish node
C. Krukenberg tumour
D. Ménétrier disease
E. Sister Mary Joseph node

F. Virchow node
G. Zollinger–Ellison syndrome
H. None of the above

For each of the following descriptions, select the most appropriate response. Each option may be used once, more than once or not at all.

1. This results from metastasis to a periumbilical lymph node.
2. This can be found in the left supraclavicular fossa as a result of metastasis.
3. This is a due to a gastric carcinoma metastasizing to the ovary.
4. This is characterized by marked gastric mucosal thickening.
5. This can be found in the left axilla as a result of metastasis.

Answers Paper 5

ANSWER QUESTION 1

1. D – Gardner syndrome
2. B – Cowden syndrome
3. E – Hereditary nonpolyposis colorectal cancer
4. C – Familial adenomatous polyposis
5. G – Peutz–Jeghers syndrome

Gardner syndrome is characterized by multiple colonic polyps and extra-colonic osteomas. The colonic polyps predispose to the development of colonic carcinoma. Cowden syndrome is a rare autosomal dominant disorder characterized by multiple hamartomas which have an increased risk of becoming malignant, especially in the breast, thyroid and uterus. In addition, up to half of all patients will suffer from a multinodular goitre. Hereditary nonpolyposis colorectal cancer is frequently caused by the mutations of the *MLH1* or *MSH2* gene. They are characterized by an increased risk of cancer due to impaired DNA mismatch repair. Familial adenomatous polyposis is an autosomal dominant condition characterised by the presence of abundant gastrointestinal polyps with malignant potential. Prophylactic colectomy is advised if more than 100 polyps are present. The patient in the final question is suffering from the autosomal dominant Peutz–Jeghers syndrome, which leads to hamartomatous polyps being present in the gastrointestinal tract. These polyps have a predisposition to cause intussusception, which is where the small intestine invaginates into another section of the small intestine and can ultimately lead to obstruction.

ANSWER QUESTION 2

1. J – SIADH
SIADH results in the uncontrolled secretion of ADH from the posterior pituitary. Causes include central nervous system (CNS) conditions, (e.g. subdural haematoma), malignancies (e.g. small cell lung cancer) and drugs, (e.g. carbamazepine). Because ADH stimulates the insertion of aquaporin II channels, the collecting duct becomes more permeable to water, and so water is conserved and urine osmolarity is high. This results in a dilutional hyponatraemia. Common presentations of SIADH

include confusion and irritability. A plasma Na⁺ concentration of less than 120 mmol/L predisposes to cerebral oedema, which can be fatal.

2. I – Spironolactone

Spironolactone is an aldosterone receptor antagonist used in congestive cardiac failure, ascites secondary to liver cirrhosis and the nephrotic syndrome. It is known as a 'potassium-sparing' diuretic, as potassium is conserved despite diuresis, predisposing to hyperkalaemia. Hyperkalaemia can cause characteristic electrocardiogram (ECG) changes, such as tall tented t waves and QRS prolongation. Severely raised potassium can result in life-threatening arrhythmias, such as ventricular tachycardia and fibrillation. Treatment must be initiated immediately and includes insulin and dextrose infusion, calcium gluconate (myocardial-protective), salbutamol nebulizers and calcium resonium.

3. A – Diabetes insipidus

Diabetes insipidus (DI) results from reduced activity of ADH. It may be cranial DI, in which ADH is not produced, or nephrogenic DI, where the kidney is not sensitive to ADH, despite it being in plentiful supply. Patients with DI are unable to produce concentrated urine in order to conserve water and so present with polydipsia, polyuria and symptoms of dehydration. Desmopressin is a synthetic ADH analogue that is effective in the management of cranial DI.

4. E – Furosemide

Furosemide is a loop diuretic that works on the Na⁺/K⁺/2Cl⁻ cotransport (NKCC) of the thick ascending limb. Along with diuresis it causes loss of potassium ions, which can result in hypokalaemia if insufficient supplementation is given. Characteristic ECG findings include flattened t waves, the presence of u waves and prolongation of the QRS interval, which predisposes to arrhythmias.

5. G – PSA

PSA is a useful screening test for prostatic carcinoma, and can be used to monitor response to treatment. However, it is a very non-specific marker and is also raised in benign prostatic hyperplasia (BPH), infections (e.g. prostatitis), and concentration rises physiologically with age. Certain procedures and examinations can elevate PSA, such as urinary catheter insertion or removal and digital rectal examination.

ANSWER QUESTION 3

1. F – Anti-tissue transglutaminase antibodies
2. B – Antigliadin antibodies
3. B – Antigliadin antibodies
4. G – Anti-topoisomerase antibodies
5. A – Antiepidermal transglutaminase

Coeliac disease serology is most specific when anti-tissue transgluta-minase antibodies are tested, although antigliadin antibodies are most specific in children under the age of 5 as it is an IgA. Systemic sclerosis is a systemic connective tissue disorder. The gastrointestinal symptoms include oesophageal dysmotility and, rarely, diverticula and pneumato-sis cystoides intestinalis. Antiepidermal transglutaminases are associ-ated with dermatitis herpetiformis, a condition associated with coeliac disease.

ANSWER QUESTION 4

1. C – Graves disease
Graves disease is the most common cause of hyperthyroidism. It is the result of auto-immunoglobulin G (IgG) antibodies against the thyroid-stimulating hormone (TSH) receptor of the thyroid gland. Symptoms of hyperthyroidism include tremor, weight loss, irritability, sweating and palpitations (e.g. with atrial fibrillation). Additional signs with Graves disease include exophthalmos, lid-lag and ophthalmoplegia. Antithyroid drugs include carbimazole and propylthiouracil, and propranolol can be used for symptomatic control.

2. I – Systemic lupus erythematosus
Systemic lupus erythematosus (SLE) is a complex multisystem disorder. Various autoantibodies can be detected in SLE but the pathogenesis is still not fully understood. Symptoms and signs can be grouped into systems, as follows:

- Nervous system: multi-infarct dementia, stroke, cranial nerve lesions, polyneuropathy
- Respiratory: pleural effusion, fibrosis
- Skin: 'butterfly' rash, purpura, photosensitivity
- Cardiovascular: pericarditis, anaemia, valvular lesions
- Musculoskeletal: myopathy, polyarthropathy
- Renal: glomerulonephritis

Corticosteroids and other disease-modifying drugs (e.g. hydroxychloro-quine) are used to manage active disease.

3. J – Type I diabetes mellitus
Type I diabetes mellitus results from self-mediated destruction of β-islet cells, leading to insulin deficiency. Diabetes usually presents in young people with the triad of polyuria, polydipsia and weight loss. Alternatively, the patient may present with ketoacidosis. Diabetic ketoacidosis results from uncontrolled catabolism in the presence of insulin deficiency. Accumulation of ketone bodies results in metabolic acidosis. The respi-ratory system tries to compensate by hyperventilating (Kussmaul respi-ration), and vomiting also occurs. Elevated glucose creates an osmotic

diuresis, which results in renal hypoperfusion, acute failure and further accumulation of ketone bodies. Fluid resuscitation and insulin are vital treatments, although care must be taken not to resuscitate too quickly, as cerebral oedema can result.

4. G – Pernicious anaemia

Pernicious anaemia is a macrocytic anaemia caused by reduced absorption of vitamin B_{12}. Parietal cell antibodies are present in around 90% of cases. However, intrinsic factor antibodies are the hallmark of the condition (although they are not detectable in all cases). Intrinsic factor is required for the absorption of B_{12} and without it macrocytic anaemia ensues. Other complications of B_{12} deficiency include optic atrophy, dementia and subacute combined degeneration of the cord. The latter presents with peripheral paraesthesia, loss of vibration sense and weakness, and can progress to ataxia and paraplegia.

5. F – Myasthenia gravis

Myasthenia gravis is a disorder of neuromuscular transmission caused by autoantibodies against acetylcholine receptors of the neuromuscular junction. Acetylcholine is unable to bind to its receptors and the clinical result is a state of muscle fatigability. Ptosis is a common sign, and muscle weakness at the end of the day illustrates the fatigable component of the disease. Acetylcholinesterase inhibitors (e.g. pyridostigmine) prevent the breakdown of acetylcholine, allowing more to be available for transmission.

ANSWER QUESTION 5

1. I – Right coronary artery

An inferior myocardial infarction occurs with occlusion of the right coronary artery. On the ECG this will show as changes in leads II, III and aVF. Management of an acute coronary syndrome includes analgesia (usually morphine and an anti-emetic), oxygen, aspirin and nitrates. An antiplatelet agent, such as clopidogrel, is given in accordance with hospital protocol. The main aim of treatment is to reperfuse the myocardium, which can occur via percutaneous coronary intervention (PCI) or thrombolysis.

2. A – Anterolateral myocardial infarction

An infarction with ST segment elevation is classified as a STEMI (ST-elevation MI). Changes in leads I, aVL and V3–6 signify an anterolateral infarction. Complications of myocardial infarction include ventricular septal defect, valvular heart disease, papillary muscle rupture, cardiac failure and arrhythmia. Prevention of coronary artery disease is important in modern practice and involves promoting a healthy lifestyle with dietary advice and exercise, smoking cessation and limiting alcohol intake.

3. B – Anterior ST-elevation myocardial infarction

The 'chest leads' are the 'V' leads. ECG changes in V1–6 signify an anterior myocardial infarction. The limb leads are I, II and III. Changes in leads II, III and aVF indicate an inferior infarction. To prevent a recurrent myocardial infarction in a patient with previous episodes, statins, angiotensin converting enzyme (ACE) inhibitors, β-blockers and antiplatelets (e.g. aspirin) are given, in addition to lifestyle advice and conservative measures.

4. K – Stable angina

Coronary artery disease is becoming increasingly common with today's sedentary lifestyles. Stable angina is a condition in which chest pain occurs on exercise, suggesting a lesser degree of atherosclerotic coronary disease, as opposed to atypical angina, which occurs at rest. Measures such as blood pressure control, cholesterol reduction, exercise, smoking cessation and diabetic control can all reduce the risk of developing coronary artery disease. Medications such as aspirin, nicorandil and diltiazem (calcium channel blocker) can be prescribed as prophylaxis.

5. H – Posterior myocardial infarction

The most commonly missed infarction is the posterior one. Reciprocal changes in the anterior leads of an ECG can indicate a posterior myocardial infarction. Classically, the R waves in V1 and 2 are large and there is ST depression. This corresponds to a STEMI in the posterior region, and treatment protocols should be commenced. Most hospital trusts have an acute coronary syndrome (ACS) protocol that guides the treatment that should be initiated. ACS includes STEMIs, NSTEMIs and unstable angina.

ANSWER QUESTION 6

1. A – Alzheimer disease

Alzheimer disease is a common neurodegenerative disorder that results in progressive dementia. Apoptosis and necrosis result in neuronal degeneration. The neurofibrillary tangles and amyloid plaques may play a role in neuronal toxicity. Episodic memory is affected early on, with gradual loss of global cognitive function, changes in behaviour and the inability to care for oneself.

2. H – Parkinson disease

Parkinson disease results in a loss of nigrostriatal dopaminergic neurones. Deposits of intraneuronal protein, called Lewy bodies, play a central role in Parkinson disease. Apoptosis and reactive oxygen species are thought to be responsible for degeneration. The disease is characterized by the triad of resting ('pill rolling') tremor, rigidity and dyskinesia. Other features include postural instability, characteristic facies and dementia. Levodopa (the dopamine precursor) is used alongside a peripheral decarboxylase inhibitor in order to prevent peripheral breakdown of L-dopa.

3. D – Huntington disease

Huntington disease is an autosomal dominant-inherited neurodegenerative disorder characterized by repeat sequences of CAG nucleotides. It usually presents in middle life with involuntary movements, chorea and dementia. There is no cure, and death usually occurs within 10–15 years. Genetic counselling is offered to the families affected.

4. F – Motor neuron disease

Motor neuron disease results in degeneration of both upper and lower motor neurones (UMN and LMN, respectively). The symptoms and signs therefore involve a mix of both, e.g. fasciculation (LMN sign) and hypertonia (UMN sign). There is widespread weakness and eventual paralysis. Wasting, cramps and fatigue are early features. Fasciculation can be seen on the tongue when there is bulbar involvement. Hyperreflexia, clonus and up-going plantars are UMN signs characteristic of the condition. Bulbar and palatal involvement results in dysphagia and dysphasia. Respiratory muscle involvement leads to respiratory failure, which is a common cause of mortality.

5. B – Creutzfeldt–Jakob disease

New variant Creutzfeldt–Jakob disease is a spongiform encephalopathy triggered by prions. Accumulation of the insoluble protein results in neurotoxicity and degeneration. It is a rapidly progressing disease resulting in loss of motor coordination, dementia and ataxia. It can be fatal within months.

ANSWER QUESTION 7

1. A – Columnar epithelium
2. B – Cuboidal epithelium
3. E – Squamous epithelium
4. E – Squamous epithelium
5. D – Pseudostratified epithelium

The basic types of epithelial tissue are squamous, cuboidal and columnar. Squamous cells are thin and flat in appearance with an elliptical nucleus. They are classically found to line surfaces at which passive diffusion occurs. Specialized squamous epithelia also line blood vessels and the heart. Cuboidal cells are cuboidal in shape. They contain a spherical nucleus and are classically found in absorptive and secretive tissue, for example the pancreas exocrine glands. Columnar cells are elongated cells with basal nuclei. Their nuclei are basal to allow for apical transfer of materials. They are found as the lining to most of the gastrointestinal tract and are interspersed with goblet cells. Transitional cells are those with a different appearance depending upon the level of stretch exerted upon them and are almost exclusively found within the bladder, urethra and ureters. 'Stratified' implies the presence of multiple layers, and stratified epithelium is consequently found where layers are abraded regularly. Pseudostratified epithelium occurs as one layer, but with nuclei at different levels within the cells.

ANSWER QUESTION 8

1. F – Positive intrapleural pressure

The pressure in the space described is called the intrapleural pressure. At baseline it is negative, preventing the lungs from collapsing. Expiration is usually a passive process, returning the intrapleural pressure to its baseline of around -4 cmH$_2$O. However, during forceful expiration, the abdominal muscles are recruited to generate a positive intrapleural pressure to force air out more quickly. In these scenarios, intrapleural pressures can rise up to $+20$ cmH$_2$O.

2. E – Negative intrapleural pressure

The pressure in the space described is called the intrapleural pressure. At rest/beginning of inspiration, intrapleural pressure is always negative due to the opposing forces created by the inherent elastic recoil of the lung pulling on the visceral pleura versus the parietal pleura fixed to the chest wall. It is about -4 cmH$_2$O. During normal inspiration, the intrapleural pressure becomes more negative and rises to around -9 cmH$_2$O. Thus, during normal inspiration, the intrapleural pressure fluctuates from about -4 to -9 cmH$_2$O.

3. G – Transmural pressure

The transmural pressure is the pressure difference, or gradient, across the walls of the lung, i.e. the difference in pressure on the inside and the outside of the lungs.

4. C – Intrapleural pressure = atmospheric pressure

The baseline negative intrapleural pressure keeps the lung held distended in the chest cavity and prevents the alveoli from collapsing. This pressure opposes the inherent elastic recoil of the lung. When intrapleural pressure equilibrates with the atmospheric pressure, for example through a communicating breach in the chest wall, the lung collapses.

5. A – Alveolar pressure

The alveolar pressure is zero at rest. At rest, alveolar pressure equals atmospheric pressure (set to zero) at baseline. When alveolar pressure equals atmospheric pressure, no airflow occurs. With negative alveolar pressure, i.e. when atmospheric pressure exceeds alveolar pressure, air flows into the lungs and vice versa.

ANSWER QUESTION 9

1. E – Diverticular disease
2. H – Pseudomembranous colitis
3. B – Carcinoma of the sigmoid colon
4. I – Ulcerative colitis
5. D – Crohn disease

Diverticular disease encompasses diverticulosis (the presence of diverticula) and diverticulitis (inflammation of diverticula). Diverticula are most common within the sigmoid colon and increase in incidence with age. It is thought that a low fibre diet and the subsequent increase in colonic pressure is the cause. The most common symptom is rectal bleeding, and diverticulitis is associated with left iliac fossa pain.

Pseudomembranous colitis is infection of the colon with *Clostridium difficile* which occurs after the use of broad-spectrum antibiotics. It is characterized by abdominal pain, fever and distinctive-smelling diarrhoea.

Ulcerative colitis is an inflammatory disease of the bowel where a patient suffers from episodes of bloody diarrhoea with mucus. There is a continuous segment of inflammation which begins in the rectum and travels proximally. Biopsy will reveal superficial ulceration. It can be cured with panproctocolectomy.

Crohn disease is an inflammatory disease of the gastrointestinal tract which may affect any part of it from the mouth to the anus. The most common sites are the terminal ileum and colon. The patient will suffer from abdominal pain, bloody diarrhoea and weight loss. There may also be extra-gastrointestinal complications such as rashes, arthritis and eye inflammation. Biopsy can be difficult as there are classically skip lesions, i.e. the inflammation is not continuous. However, if correctly biopsied, granulomatous transmural inflammation/ulceration will be demonstrated.

ANSWER QUESTION 10

1. G – Nifedipine
Nifedipine is a calcium channel blocker. In vascular smooth muscle, nifedipine causes a reduction of influx of calcium into the cell and thus a reduction in the concentration of intracellular calcium, resulting in reduced muscle contraction. Vasodilation is the consequence. Calcium channel blockers work on the heart as well as vascular smooth muscle to varying degrees. Dihydropyridines like nifedipine work well on vascular smooth muscle.

2. H – Nitroprusside
Once in the bloodstream, nitroprusside undergoes metabolism to release nitric oxide (NO), which works on the endothelium to cause

vasodilation in the arteries and veins. It is used as an intravenous drug in hypertensive emergencies.

3. F – Nicorandil
Nicorandil is a potassium channel activator. This hyperpolarizes vascular smooth muscle cells and relaxes them, causing vasodilation. Note that nicorandil also works by donating NO to guanylate cyclase. Both these mechanisms lead to vasodilation.

4. D – Doxazosin
Sympathetic vasoconstriction is mediated by alpha-1 adrenoceptors. As such, selective alpha-1 antagonists such as doxazosin can inhibit vasoconstriction and treat hypertension.

5. B – Candesartan
Angiotensin II is a potent vasoconstrictor and acts via the AT1 (angiotensin II subtype 1) receptor. Drugs like candesartan are AT1 antagonists and thus are vasodilators by inhibiting vasoconstriction. AT1 antagonists can be used instead of angiotensin-converting enzyme (ACE) inhibitors if ACE inhibitors are not tolerated by patients because of their side effects, e.g. dry cough.

ANSWER QUESTION 11

1. B – Adrenalectomy
In cases where there is a benign unilateral tumour, adrenalectomy is curative and can be performed laparoscopically. Bilateral hyperplasia is usually managed with spironolactone, which helps both in controlling the blood pressure and normalizing potassium concentrations.

2. H – Spironolactone
Spironolactone preoperatively controls blood pressure and raises potassium levels. Side-effects include gynaecomastia in men. An alternative aldosterone antagonist, eplerenone, does not cause gynaecomastia so frequently, but it is licensed only for left ventricular failure post-myocardial infarction.

3. D – Dexamethasone
Glucocorticoid-remediable aldosteronism is inherited in an autosomal dominant fashion. Glucocorticoids are used to suppress ACTH secretion. This does not always normalize blood pressure but is usually effective in regulating biochemistry.

4. E – Eplerenone
Eplerenone is a selective aldosterone receptor antagonist.

5. G – Renal artery stenosis
Renal artery stenosis leads to reduced perfusion of the kidneys and an increase in renin levels, and thus to aldosterone secretion.

ANSWER QUESTION 12

1. C – Complete heart block

This patient has sustained an extensive anterior MI and has now developed complete heart block. It is important to understand intrinsic nodal rates to understand the physiology behind this. The sinoatrial node has an intrinsic pacemaker rate of between 60 and 100 per minute. The atrioventricular node controls the rate at which ventricular contraction occurs and has an intrinsic firing rate of 40–60 per minute. In complete heart block there is complete atrioventricular dissociation which results in both the ventricles and atria pacing at their own intrinsic rates.

2. D – Dressler syndrome

This is the typical time frame for Dressler syndrome to occur, which can develop from 2 to 10 weeks post MI or heart surgery. The cause is thought to be the formation of autoantibodies directed against cardiac myocytes. Treatment is with non-steroidal anti-inflammatory agents and steroids.

3. E – Left ventricular failure

This patient has developed left ventricular failure, which is a relatively common complication of lateral infarcts. An echocardiogram is likely to show a reduced left ventricular ejection fraction with regional wall motion abnormalities.

4. A – Atrial fibrillation

Atrial fibrillation has complicated this MI. Atrial fibrillation is the most common cardiac arrhythmia encountered. Management should be targeted at either rate or rhythm control. It is important to remember that patients will require some form of anticoagulation. This may be with warfarin or aspirin if warfarin is contraindicated or the patient is at low risk of emboli. In the acute setting, heparin may be more appropriate.

5. H – Ventricular tachycardia

This patient has developed ventricular tachycardia. She has become decompensated and unwell with this and requires urgent management. A peri-arrest call/arrest call for this patient should be put out and help requested. She is likely to require DC cardioversion. If she is stable and well with this, it may be possible to chemically cardiovert her.

ANSWER QUESTION 13

1. F – Sphenoid sinus
2. A – Ethmoid air cells
3. E – Maxillary sinus
4. B – Frontal sinus
5. C – Mastoid cells

The sphenoidal sinus arises from the nasal capsule of the embryonic nose, as opposed to the other paranasal sinuses which arise from outpouchings of the nasal cavity. The ethmoid air cells are more variable in their location and can be found above the orbit, lateral to the sphenoid and within the roof of the maxillary sinus. This variability means preoperative imaging is essential for sinus surgery. The maxillary sinus contains the highest density of goblet cells for the production of mucus. Cholesteatoma is a destructive and expanding keratinizing squamous epithelium in the mastoid process. It can lead to hearing loss.

ANSWER QUESTION 14

1. A – Axillary nerve
Shoulder dislocation most commonly (95%) occurs in the antero-inferior direction. Because the axillary nerve courses close to the inferior margin of the head of the humerus and then winds around its surgical neck, it is prone to damage in glenohumeral dislocations. Axillary nerve palsy affects the deltoid, teres minor and the long head of the triceps. Its superior lateral cutaneous branch supplies sensation to a small area of skin on the inferior edge of the deltoid. This corresponds to the regimental badge on a military uniform.

2. H – Sciatic nerve
The hip joint is a ball-and-socket joint with the ability to move in any plane. It is relatively stable, with a deep acetabulum and pubofemoral, ischiofemoral and iliofemoral ligaments to strengthen the joint. However, trauma or congenital abnormality can lead to dislocation, which most commonly occurs in the posterior direction. The close relationship of the sciatic nerve to the hip joint makes it vulnerable to damage in posterior dislocation. This can present with pain along the posterior aspect of the leg, with weakness of the hip extensors or knee flexors. Weakness of inversion and plantar flexion may also result.

3. G – Radial nerve
The radial nerve courses along the radial groove of the humerus. A fracture of the humeral shaft can result in damage to the radial nerve. This classically presents as weakness of the forearm extensors (i.e. wrist drop). Because of the overlap of sensory supply in the hand, radial nerve damage results in the loss of only a small amount of sensation over the first web space on the dorsum of the hand.

4. D – Median nerve
Carpal tunnel syndrome results in compression of the median nerve as it passes between the carpal bones and flexor retinaculum. Conditions predisposing to carpal tunnel syndrome include rheumatoid arthritis, pregnancy, acromegaly, hypothyroidism and diabetes. The median nerve

supplies the muscles of the thenar eminence and sensation to the lateral three-and-a-half digits.

5. C – Lateral cutaneous nerve

Weight change can cause meralgia paraesthetica (or Bernhardt–Roth syndrome). The lateral cutaneous nerve of the thigh is compressed along its course, commonly between the inguinal ligament and ileum. This presents as loss of sensation or pain on the lateral thigh. It is thought that weight gain may cause compression of the nerve by clothing, underwear or belts. Weight loss can remove protective fat pads that cushion and protect the nerve.

ANSWER QUESTION 15

1. F – Koilonychia
2. C – Erythroplakia
3. D – Glossitis
4. H – Leukoplakia
5. E – Hairy leukoplakia

Koilonychia is associated with iron deficiency anaemia. Erythroplakia is associated with squamous cell carcinoma. Glossitis is the inflammation of the tongue – the papillae may be lost and the tongue may appear smooth. It is associated with pernicious anaemia. Leukoplakia is a premalignant condition primarily caused by the use of tobacco. Hairy leukoplakia is seen in those severely immunocompromised and is caused by the Epstein–Barr virus. Angular cheilitis is an inflammatory lesion at the corner of the mouth. It may occur in patients with zinc deficiency and Plummer–Vinson syndrome. An apthous ulcer is an oral ulcer and is commonly seen in Crohn disease. Leukonychia is a white discolouration of the nail, and while often due to trauma, it can also be a sign of hypoalbuminaemia.

ANSWER QUESTION 16

1. D – Haemorrhage

The causes of renal failure are divided into three groups: pre-renal, intrinsic and post-renal. Pre-renal failure occurs as a result of impaired renal perfusion. This can be caused by haemorrhage, sepsis or dehydration, causing hypovolaemia. Poor renal perfusion may be exacerbated by drugs such as diuretics, non-steroidal anti-inflammatory drugs (NSAIDs) and angiotensin-converting enzyme (ACE) inhibitors. Pre-renal failure can occur secondary to cardiac failure because of reduced cardiac output and resultant hypotension.

2. H – Renal calculi

Post-renal failure results from obstruction of the urinary tract at any point distal to the renal calyces. Causes include benign prostatic hyperplasia in men, renal calculi, pelvic tumours causing compression of the urinary tract and ureteric strictures. Urinary tract obstruction is investigated using ultrasonography.

3. E – Polycystic kidney disease

Polycystic kidney disease (PCKD) is an autosomal dominant disorder resulting in multiple renal cysts and progressive renal failure. It is the most commonly inherited nephropathy in the Western world. Acute episodes present with haematuria and pain. PCKD is associated with multiple other pathologies including hepatic cysts, renal calculi, hypertension and subarachnoid haemorrhage. Subarachnoid haemorrhage carries a high mortality rate and occurs as a result of rupture of berry aneurysms, presenting with a 'thunderclap' headache, vomiting and reduced consciousness.

4. I – Renal cell carcinoma

Renal cell carcinoma arises from epithelial cells of the proximal convoluted tubule. It is characterized by haematuria, loin pain and a ballotable mass, along with systemic symptoms of malignancy (e.g. weight loss, malaise, fever). Renal cell carcinoma metastasizes to the brain, bone, liver and lungs. Pulmonary metastases are commonly seen as 'cannonball metastases' on the chest X-ray and patients may present with progressive dyspnoea, reduced exercise tolerance and haemoptysis.

5. J – Tubular necrosis

Aminoglycosides, such as gentamicin, are nephrotoxic and cause tubular necrosis, which can result in intrinsic renal failure. Gentamicin is indicated for the treatment of sepsis, meningitis, biliary tract infection and hospital-acquired pneumonia. In addition to its effects on the kidney, gentamicin is ototoxic and can cause colitis and stomatitis. Regular gentamicin monitoring is required to assess plasma concentrations to ensure that the drug is within the therapeutic range without reaching toxic levels. Hospital protocols and the British National Formulary should be consulted to ensure that a safe dosing regimen is being followed.

ANSWER QUESTION 17

1. I – Surgery

Surgery, infection, trauma or forgetting steroid tablets when on long-term treatment can all lead to an Addisonian crisis. The stress of surgery on the body requires an appropriate stress response. Anaesthetists will usually increase the dose of steroids for the perioperative period.

2. G – Hypoglycaemia

Hypoglycaemia occurs during an Addisonian crisis and may be the presenting complaint with related clinical signs/symptoms.

3. B – Fluid resuscitation

The initial management of shock should always begin with examining airway, breathing and circulation. When the diagnosis of an Addisonian crisis has been made, fluid resuscitation should begin along with replacement of steroids.

4. C – Hydrocortisone IV

An Addisonian crisis is potentially fatal if treatment is not initiated promptly. IV fluids and hydrocortisone must be commenced immediately if a crisis is suspected. Hypotension and severe pain in the abdomen or back are common signs of a crisis. Loss of consciousness will follow if treatment is not administered. Exogenous steroids must be given to takeover the lack of endogenous production.

5. F – Hyperpigmentation of palmar creases

Increased levels of adrenocorticotrophic hormone (ACTH) lead to hyperpigmentation of the palmar creases and buccal mucosa. ACTH is formed from the precursor POMC (pro-opimelanocortin). Melanin is also cleaved from POMC and so its excess leads to increased levels of melanin, and thus hyperpigmentation.

ANSWER QUESTION 18

1. C – Reticulospinal tract

The reticulospinal tract controls locomotion and postural control. It controls the proximal parts of the limbs and trunk in walking.

2. G – Vestibulospinal tract

The vestibulospinal tract maintains the centre of gravity between the feet. It controls the reflexes that alter body position in relation to movements of the head.

3. B – Raphespinal tract

The raphespinal tracts are serotoninergic fibres which are involved in the inhibition of transmission of nociceptive information through the dorsal horn.

4. F – Tectospinal tract

The tectospinal tract is postulated to be associated with head and trunk orientation following visual and auditory stimuli.

5. D – Spinocerebellar tract

The spinocerebellar tract conveys information to the cerebellum about limb and joint position obtained from the golgi tendon organs and muscle spindles.

ANSWER QUESTION 19

1. I – Z-lines
2. B – Actin

3. F – Myosin
4. C – Actinin
5. B – Actin

Skeletal muscle fibres consist of several smaller subunits called myofibrils. These myofibrils are a series of parallel subunits that contain the contractile proteins of the skeletal muscle fibre. When looked at closely myofibrils have a banded appearance, consisting of light and dark bands. The light bands are called I-bands and consist of thin myofilaments. The dark bands are called A-bands and are made up of thick myofilaments. The Z-line is a line which dissects each I-band. The interval between two adjacent Z-lines is called a sarcomere and a sarcomere is a basic contractile unit of skeletal muscle.

Z-lines contain a protein called α (alpha) actinin. Alpha-actinin anchors the thin myofilaments of the skeletal muscle fibre. Thin myofilaments are small, measuring 5 nm in width and 1 μm in length. Thick myofilaments are larger than thin myofilaments and they measure 10 nm in width and 1.5 μm in length. Thick myofilaments lie between the thin myofilaments. The partial interdigitation between the thin myofilaments and the thick myofilaments is what gives the appearance of the light and dark bands which give striated skeletal muscle its name. Light 'I' bands are portions of actin which do not overlap with myosin. Dark 'A' bands, on the other hand, represent the filaments of actin which overlap with the myosin filaments. During the contraction of a sarcomere, the 'I' band shortens but the 'A' band's length remains unchanged.

ANSWER QUESTION 20

1. E – Sister Mary Joseph node
2. F – Virchow node
3. C – Krukenberg tumour
4. D – Ménétrier disease
5. B – Irish node

A Krukenberg tumour is a metastasis from the gastrointestinal tract to the ovary. A Sister Mary Joseph node is a metastasis to a periumbilical lymph node. Virchow node is found following metastasis from the stomach to the left supraclavicular node. Irish node metastasis is from the stomach to the left axillary node. Ménétrier disease is also known as giant hypertrophic gastropathy and is a rare disease characterized by marked gastric mucosal fold thickening, hypersecretion, hypochlorhydria and hypoproteinaemia. The Carman meniscus sign is created by a large, flat gastric ulcer with heaped-up edges. The edges of the ulcer trap a lenticular barium collection that is convex relative to the lumen when the edges are folded upon themselves during compression. These findings are indicative of a malignant gastric ulcer.

Index

Milton Keynes UK
Ingram Content Group UK Ltd.
UKHW031152141024
449569UK00024B/868